THE INTERNAL MEDICINE COMPANION

THE
INTERNAL MEDICINE
COMPANION

FRED F. FERRI, M.D., F.A.C.P.

Clinical Assistant Professor
Department of Medicine
Brown University
Chief, Division of Internal Medicine
St. Joseph's Hospital
Providence, Rhode Island

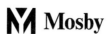

St. Louis Baltimore Boston Chicago London Madrid Philadelphia Sydney Toronto

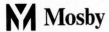

Mosby

Dedicated to Publishing Excellence

Publisher: George Stamathis
Acquisition Editor: Stephanie Manning
Developmental Editor: Kathy Falk
Project Manager: Gayle May Morns
Production Editor: Mary Cusick Drone
Manufacturing Supervisor: Theresa Fuchs
Designer: Susan Lane

Cover Image: "The Doctor," by Sir Luke Fildes (1844-1927).
            Detail
            Tate Gallery, London/Art Resource, NY.

Printed in the United States of America
Composition by The Clarinda Company
Printing/binding by R.R. Donnelley & Sons Company

Mosby–Year Book, Inc.
11830 Westline Industrial Drive
St. Louis, Missouri 63146

International Standard Book Number 0-8016-7825-0

93 94 95 96 97 / 9 8 7 6 5 4 3 2 1

With the publication of its fourth edition, Stein's *Internal Medicine* has become *the* reference text for medical students, residents and practicing physicians. Its authors have successfully written a textbook that is up-to-date, readable and encyclopedic.

I have attempted to extract its salient points (i.e., important things one forgets to remember) and to combine them in a practical companion handbook which can be conveniently carried in a coat pocket.

To limit its size I have avoided an encyclopedic approach and focused on selected topics. Medical tables and figures are used throughout the handbook to enhance recollection of key points. In order to follow a logical and practical approach, the information has been subdivided in to the following eight parts:

Etiology of common diseases
Differential diagnosis
Classification of disease processes
Diagnostic approach
Therapeutic modalities
Medication comparison tables
Laboratory evaluation
Appendix

The reader is encouraged to use this handbook as a temporary extension of Stein's *Internal Medicine* text and subsequently review that particular topic in the main text as time permits.

FRED F. FERRI

PART TWO
Differential Diagnosis

PART THREE
Classification of Disease Processes

PART FOUR
Diagnostic Approach

PART FIVE
Therapeutic Modalities

PART SIX
Medication Comparison Tables

PART SEVEN
Laboratory Evaluation

PART EIGHT
Appendix

Etiology of Common Diseases

Causes of chronic abdominal pain

  I. Inflammatory causes
    A. Chronic pancreatitis
    B. Pelvic inflammatory disease
    C. Crohn's disease
    D. Chronic ulcerative colitis
    E. Tuberculous peritonitis
    F. Chronic cholecystitis
 II. Neoplastic causes
    A. Adenocarcinoma of pancreas
    B. Carcinoma of stomach
    C. Carcinomatosis peritonei
    D. Primary hepatocellular carcinoma
    E. Mesothelioma of peritoneum
    F. Carcinoma of kidney
    G. Intra-abdominal or retroperitoneal lymphoma
    H. Carcinoma of ovary
III. Metabolic causes
    A. Porphyria
    B. Lead poisoning
    C. Adrenal insufficiency
 IV. Vascular causes
    A. Aortic aneurysm
    B. Mesenteric vascular insufficiency ("abdominal angina")
  V. Other causes
    A. Irritable bowel syndrome
    B. Distended urinary bladder
    C. Fecal impaction
    D. Hydronephrosis
    E. Mesenteric cyst
    F. Endometriosis
    G. Ovarian cyst
    H. Psychogenic

Metabolic acidosis

Anion gap present

Ketoacidosis
  Diabetic ketoacidosis
  Alcoholic ketoacidosis
  Starvation ketoacidosis
Lactic acidosis
Methanol ingestion
Salicylate ingestion
Paraldehyde ingestion
Ethylene glycol ingestion
Uremic acidosis

Anion gap not present

Diarrhea
Pancreato-cutaneous fistula
Mineral acid ingestion
Hyperalimentation
Renal acidosis
  Proximal renal tubular acidosis
  Distal renal tubular acidosis
    Hypokalemic
      Pump failure
      Acid backleak
    Hyperkalemic
      "Short-circuit acidosis" (voltage
        dependent)
      Aldosterone deficiency or resis-
        tance
      Addison's disease
      Hyporeninemic-
        hypoaldosteronism
Renal failure with volume contraction

Causes of respiratory acidosis

Disorders of ventilatory control
   Central nervous system
      Depression of respiratory center
         Anesthetics
         Drug intoxication
         Primary central hypoventilation
         Myxedema
         Oxygen therapy in chronic hypercapnic patients
         Sleep
   Peripheral neuromuscular disease
      Disorders of peripheral nerves
         Spinal cord injury
         Phrenic nerve palsy
         Guillain-Barré syndrome
         Myasthenia gravis
         Paralytic agents
         Botulism
      Disorders of muscle
         Myositis, myopathy, muscular dystrophies
         Fatigue in hypokalemia, hypophosphatemia
         Fatigue in obstructive airways disease
Disorders of pulmonary function
   Restrictive lung disease
      Kyphoscoliosis
      Flail chest
   Airways obstruction
      Upper airways obstruction (trachea, larynx, bronchi)
      Asthma and chronic obstructive pulmonary disease
Shunts
   Congenital heart disease with left to right shunt
   Intrapulmonary shunt
      Arteriovenous malformation
      Severe pneumonia, large emboli
Errors of ventilator management

Causes of adrenocortical insufficiency

Primary adrenocortical insufficiency
    Acquired disorders (Addison's disease)
        Idiopathic autoimmunity
        Infectious causes (tuberculosis, AIDS, fungal infections, sepsis)
        Metastic or invasive disorder (tumors, sarcoidosis, amyloidosis)
        Adrenal hemorrhage (trauma, shock, coagulopathies)
        Iatrogenic (surgery, adrenal inhibitors, anticoagulation)
    Congenital and familial
        Congenital adrenal hyperplasia (enzymatic deficiencies)
        Congenital adrenal hypoplasia
        Congenital unresponsiveness to ACTH
        Adrenoleukodystrophy
        Adrenomyeloneuropathy
Secondary adrenocortical insufficiency
    Hypothalamopituitary suppression by glucocorticoids
        Exogenous glucocorticoid or ACTH administration
        Endogenous suppression by adrenal or pituitary hyperfunction
            (Cushing's syndrome)
    Hypothalamopituitary disease
        Invasive neoplasms (pituitary tumor, craniopharyngioma, eosi-
            nophilic granuloma, lymphoma, leukemia)
        Infections (tuberculosis, fungal)
        Surgery and trauma

Metabolic alkalosis

Generation

Loss of acid
  Gastrointestinal losses
    Vomiting
    Chloride-losing diarrhea of
      infancy
  Renal losses
    Increased acid excretion due
      to aldosterone excess
      Secondary hyperaldoste-
        ronism
        All causes of volume
          loss, diuretics
      Primary aldosteronism
        Conn's syndrome
        Cushing's syndrome
      Pseudohyperaldoster-
        onism
        Liddle's syndrome
        Bartter's syndrome
        Licorice ingestion
Ingestion of alkali
  Absorbable antacids
    "Milk alkali" syndrome
  Absorbable bicarbonate pre-
    cursors
    Lactate, citrate, acetate
  Intravenous alkali
    Bicarbonate administra-
      tion
    Acetate in dialysis

Maintenance

Volume depletion
  Diminished filtered load of
    bicarbonate
  Diminished distal delivery
Role of potassium
Role of chloride?

Causes of respiratory alkalosis

Hypoxemia
  Most pulmonary disease
  Organic heart disease
    Congenital heart disease with right to left shunts
    Congestive heart failure
  Altitude
Stimulation of respiratory center
  Drugs
    Salicylates
    Catecholamines
    Theophylline
    Nikethemide, ethmivan, doxapram
  Progesterone excess
    Pregnancy
    Cirrhosis
  CNS disease
    Subarachnoid hemorrhage
    Disease of respiratory center
    Cheyne-Stokes respirations
  Fever
  Sepsis
  Anxiety
Stimulation of peripheral pulmonary receptors
  Pneumonia
  Asthma
  Embolism
  Pulmonary edema
  Pulmonary fibrosis
  Pleural disease
Errors of ventilator management

Causes of amnesia

Cerebrovascular events
  Hippocampal lesions
  Thalamic lesions
  Basal forebrain lesions
Wernicke-Korsakoff syndrome
Head trauma
Hypoxia
Hypoglycemia
Herpes simplex encephalitis
Degenerative diseases
  Alzheimer's disease
  Pick's disease
  Huntington's disease
Creutzfeldt-Jakob disease
Transient global amnesia
Neoplasms
Limbic encephalitis
Postsurgery
  Bilateral temporal lobectomy
  Bilateral fornix section
  Mammillary body surgery
  Cingulectomy

Etiology of iron deficiency anemia

I. Blood loss
   A. Menstrual
   B. Gastrointestinal
      1. Stomach
         a. Hiatal hernia
         b. Esophageal varices
         c. Peptic ulcer disease
         d. Acute gastritis
         e. Drugs
         f. Carcinoma of the stomach
      2. Large bowel
         a. Carcinoma of the colon/rectum
         b. Benign polyps
         c. Angiodysplasia
         d. Diverticular disease
         e. Ulcerative colitis
      3. Small bowel
         a. Hookworm
         b. Crohn's disease
         c. Milk allergy
   C. Other
      1. Epistaxis
      2. Hematuria
      3. Coagulopathy
      4. Blood donation
      5. Chronic hemodialysis
II. Malabsorption
   A. Achlorhydria
   B. Total gastrectomy
   C. Gastrojejunostomy
   D. Celiac disease and spruelike syndromes
   E. Pica
III. Inadequate intake or increased requirements
   A. Dietary (rare)
   B. Pregnancy and lactation
   C. Growth and development
IV. Miscellaneous
   A. Pulmonary sequestration of iron (Goodpasture's syndrome)
   B. Hemosiderinuria

Pathogenesis of constipation

1. Decreased fecal water content
   a. Dehydration
   b. Decreased oral intake
   c. Decreased bulk intake
2. Obstruction to flow
   a. Ileal
      (1) Constipation by prevention of normal passage of intraluminal contents
      (2) Presents with signs and symptoms of small bowel obstruction
   b. Colonic
      (1) Extraluminal (diverticular abscess, adhesions, distended urinary bladder, mesenteric tumor, etc.)
      (2) Intramural (intramural hematoma, etc.)
      (3) Intraluminal (carcinoma, polyp, intussusception, etc.)
   c. Anal
      (1) Extraluminal (fibrosis, etc.)
      (2) Intraluminal (tumors, etc.)
3. Decreased or altered motility
   a. Generalized (may present as acute ileus)
      (1) Drugs (opiates)
      (2) Hypothyroidism and other metabolic disorders
      (3) Intestinal pseudo-obstruction
      (4) Scleroderma, progressive systemic sclerosis
      (5) Diabetic enteropathy
      (6) Spinal cord injury (lumbosacral cord, paraplegia)
      (7) Bed rest
   b. Colonic: Irritable bowel syndrome
4. Altered defecation reflex
   a. Hirschsprung's disease (short segment in adults)
   b. Secondary to painful rectal or anal lesions
   c. Other causes of idiopathic constipation associated with abnormal anal manometric findings
   d. Psychiatric illness

Causes of acute confusional state

Metabolic dysfunction
  Electrolyte abnormalities
  Hepatic failure
  Renal failure
  Hypoxia
  Hypercarbia
  Endocrinopathies (e.g., thyroid, parathyroid, and adrenal dysfunction)
  Blood glucose abnormalities
  Acidosis
  Alkalosis
  Porphyria
  Vitamin deficiencies
Drugs and toxins
  Psychoactive medications
  Alcohol
  Toxic ingestions
  Drug and alcohol withdrawal
Infections
  Systemic infections
  CNS infections (meningitis, encephalitis)
Seizures
  Complex partial seizures
  Psychomotor and absence status epilepticus
  Postictal states
Brain disease
  Focal brain lesions
    Right parietal lobe
    Medial occipital lobes
    Right frontal lobe
  Generalized brain lesions
    Head trauma
    Hypertensive encephalopathy
    Subdural hematoma
    Space-occupying masses
    Vasculitis
    Petechial hemorrhages

Causes of diabetes insipidus

I. Vasopressin deficiency (neurogenic or central diabetes insipidus)
  A. Decreased secretion
    1. Idiopathic
      a. Sporadic (? autoimmune)
      b. Familial (autosomal dominant inheritance)
    2. Traumatic (accidental or surgical)
    3. Malignancy
      a. Primary (craniopharyngioma, germinoma, meningi-
         oma, pituitary adenoma with suprasellar extension)
      b. Metastatic (lung, breast, leukemia)
    4. Granuloma (sarcoid, histiocytosis, xanthoma dissemina-
       tion)
    5. Infectious (meningitis, encephalitis, syphilis)
    6. Vascular (aneurysm, Sheehan's syndrome, cardiac arrest,
       vasculitis)
    7. Psychobiologic (anorexia nervosa)
    8. Toxic (carbon monoxide)
    9. Congenital malformations
  B. Increased metabolism
    1. Pregnancy
II. Vasopressin resistance (nephrogenic diabetes insipidus)
  A. Idiopathic
    1. Sporadic
    2. Familial (X-linked recessive inheritance)
  B. Post obstructive
  C. Malignancy (retroperitoneal fibrosarcoma)
  D. Granuloma (sarcoid)
  E. Infectious (pyelonephritis)
  F. Vascular (sickle cell disease or trait)
  G. Metabolic (hypokalemia, hypercalciuria)
  H. Toxic (lithium, demeclocycline, methoxyflurane, methicillin)
  I. Malformations (polycystic disease)
  J. Pregnancy
III. Excessive water intake (primary polydipsia)
  A. Psychogenic (schizophrenia, affective disorders)
  B. Dipsogenic
    1. Idiopathic
    2. Traumatic
    3. Granuloma (neurosarcoidosis)
    4. Infectious (meningitis)
    5. Other (multiple sclerosis)

Causes of diffuse (disseminated) intravascular coagulation (DIC)

Obstetric complications

Amniotic fluid embolism
Abruptio placentae
Retained dead fetus
Eclampsia
Septic abortion
Induced abortion
Hydatidiform mole

Shock

Hemorrhagic
Traumatic
Septic
Anaphylactic

Carcinoma

Prostate
Lung
Pancreas
Stomach
Ovary
Colon
Sarcoma

Infections

Bacterial (gram positive and
    negative)
Viral (herpes)
Rickettsial (Rocky Mountain
    spotted fever)
Fungal (aspergillosis)
Parasitic (malaria)
Granulomatous (tuberculosis)

Vascular and pulmonary

Pulmonary embolism
Hyaline membrane disease
Crush syndrome
Malignant hypertension
Cardiopulmonary bypass pump
Thoracic surgery
Giant hemangioma
Fat embolism

Hematologic

Promyelocytic leukemia
Acute leukemia
Tranfusion reaction
Acquired hemolytic anemia
Sickle cell crisis

Renal

Transplant rejection
Glomerulonephritis
Acute renal failure

Miscellaneous

Hepatic cirrhosis
Acute pancreatitis
Allergic drug reaction
Snakebite
Decompression sickness
Amyloidosis
Heatstroke

Causes of generalized edema

I. Common causes
   A. Congestive heart failure
   B. Cirrhosis of the liver
   C. Nephrotic syndrome
   D. Acute "nephritic" syndrome
   E. Pregnancy
      1. Normal pregnancy
      2. Toxemia of pregnancy
   F. Idiopathic edema
II. Unusual causes
   A. Arteriovenous fistulas
   B. Hypothyroidism
   C. Diabetes mellitus
      1. Associated with microangiopathy (rare)
      2. Associated with insulin treatment of ketoacidosis
   D. Drugs
      1. Nonsteroidal anti-inflammatory drugs
      2. Estrogens
      3. Vasodilator antihypertensive drugs
      4. Hyperstimulation syndrome secondary to menotropins (Pergonal)

Cardiogenic sources of emboli

Myocardial ischemia
   Mural thrombi
   Hypokinetic zones
   Ventricular aneurysms
Arrhythmia
   Atrial fibrillation (especially recent or paroxysmal)
   Sick sinus syndrome
Valvular
   Bacterial or marantic endocarditis
   Rheumatic mitral or aortic stenosis
   Bicuspid aortic valve
   Mitral valve prolapse
   Calcific aortic stenosis
   Mitral annulus calcification
Cardiomyopathies
   Endocardial fibroelactosis
   Alcoholic cardiomyopathy
   Myocarditis
   Amyloid
Intracardiac lesions
   Myxomas
   Primary or metastatic cardiac malignancies
   Ball valve thrombi
Intracardiac defects with paradoxic emboli
   Atrial septal defects
   Patent foramen ovale

Causes of acute metabolic encephalopathy

I. Substrate deficiency
   Hypoxia/ischemia
   Hypoglycemia
   Carbon monoxide poisoning
   Hypoxia
II. Cofactor deficiency
   Thiamin
   Vitamin B_{12}
   Pyridoxine (isoniazid administration)
III. Electrolyte disorders
   Hyponatremia
   Hypercalcemia
   CO_2 narcosis
   Dialysis disequilibrium syndrome
IV. Endocrinopathies
   Diabetes
      Ketoacidosis
      Nonketotic hyperglycemic hyperosmolar coma
   Thyroid
   Adrenal
   Parathyroid
V. Endogenous toxins
   Liver disease
      Portal-systemic shunting
      Liver failure
   Uremia
   Porphyria
   Subarachnoid hemorrhage
VI. Exogenous toxins
   Drug overdose
      Sedative/hypnotics
      Ethanol
      Narcotics
      Salicylates
      Tricyclic antidepressants
   Industrial toxins (e.g., organophosphorus insecticides, heavy
      metals)
   Meningitis
   Sepsis
VII. Heat stroke
VIII. Epilepsy (postictal)
IX. Drug withdrawal

Causes of eosinophilia and basophilia

I. Eosinophilia
   A. Metazoan infestation, especially amebiasis, ascariasis, schisto-somiasis, strongyloidiasis, trichinosis, visceral larva migrans
   B. Allergic conditions: bronchial asthma, allergic rhinitis, eczema, acute allergic reactions to drugs or food, insect bites
   C. Skin diseases: especially atopic dermatitis, acute urticaria, pemphigus, pemphigoid, eczema
   D. Pulmonary eosinophilias: tropical eosinophilia, visceral larva migrans, ascariasis, fungal infections, inhalation of allergens, Churg-Strauss allergic granulomatosis
   E. Neoplastic diseases: acute myelogenous leukemia, Hodgkin's and non-Hodgkin's lymphomas, solid tumors, especially carcinoma of the lung
   F. Immunologic disorders: polyarteritis nodosa, rheumatoid arthritis, angioimmunoblastic lymphadenopathy
   G. Idiopathic hypereosinophilic syndrome
II. Basophilia
   A. Allergic conditions: drugs, foods, inhalants
   B. Myeloproliferative disorders
   C. Miscellaneous conditions: myxedema, ulcerative colitis, systemic mast cell disease
   D. Basophilic leukemia

Common causes of acute glomerulonephritis

I. Hypocomplementemic glomerulonephritis
   A. Primary renal diseases
      1. Acute poststreptococcal glomerulonephritis
      2. Membranoproliferative glomerulonephritis
   B. Systemic diseases
      1. Systemic lupus erythematosus
      2. Infectious endocarditis
      3. Ventriculoatrial shunt infection associated nephritis
      4. Cryoglobulinemia
II. Normocomplementemic glomerulonephritis
   A. Primary renal diseases
      1. IgA nephritis
      2. Idiopathic rapidly progressive glomerulonephritis
      3. Antiglomerular basement membrane disease
   B. Systemic diseases
      1. Vasculitis (e.g., Wegener's granulomatosis, polyarteritis nodosa, hypersensitivity vasculitis)
      2. Goodpasture syndrome
      3. Henoch-Schönlein purpura
      4. Others (e.g., hemolytic-uremic syndrome, thrombotic thrombocytopenic purpura, visceral abscesses)

Modified from Madaio M and Harrington JT: N Engl J Med 309:1299-1302, 1983.

Glomerulonephritis, acute

Causes of gynecomastia

Cause	Mechanisms and clinical features
Physiologic	
Puberty	Gonadotropin stimulation of the prepubertal testis initially produces estradiol secretion. Later, testosterone secretion is dominant and gynecomastia is consequently transient
Senescence	Uncertain mechanisms but probably related to decreased serum levels, testosterone and increased sex hormone-binding globulin (TeBG) resulting in a reduction in biologically available testosterone
Pathologic	
Hypogonadism	Reduced testosterone secretion. Estrogens from the adrenal and from peripheral conversion of andro-
Primary testicular disease or secondary to hypothalamic-pituitary disorders	stenedione produce a relative estrogen excess. Gynecomastia is usually present in Klinefelter's syndrome and less commonly in hypothalamic-pituitary disease
Androgen-resistance syndromes	Abnormalities of the cytosolic androgen receptor, which is absent in testicular feminization and is re-
Testicular feminization, complete and partial forms; Reifenstein's syndrome	duced in number or has abnormal function in partial syndromes. Testosterone action is absent or reduced. Elevated LH and FSH levels stimulate testosterone and estradiol secretion, but only estradiol has peripheral effects. Gynecomastia is usually present. The phenotype may be female in testicular feminization, and varying degrees of abnormal scrotal fusion or hypospadias are present in partial forms
Tumors	
Testicular—Leydig's cell	Estradiol secreted by Leydig's cell tumors
Teratoma or choriocarcinoma	hCG secretion may be present

Adrenal	Some adrenal carcinomas secrete estradiol
Other—adenocarcinomas of lung and stomach, hepatoblastomas	Secretion of gonadotropins or hCG by tumors
Starvation and refeeding	Weight loss caused by starvation, malabsorption, or chronic illness is associated with gonadotropin-releasing hormone (GnRH) deficiency. With recovery, GnRH secretion increases, hormonal changes resemble those seen in normal puberty, and transient gynecomastia may occur
Hyperthyroidism	Mechanisms uncertain. Thyroid hormones increase TeBG synthesis, and testosterone binding is increased. Peripheral conversion of androgens to estrogen is increased and leads to a relative estrogen excess
Cirrhosis	Reduced estradiol metabolism. Increased serum estrogen concentrations suppress LH and FSH levels and also increase TeBG levels. Testosterone binding is increased, and a state of relative estrogen excess results
Renal failure	Mechanisms are uncertain, but serum testosterone level is reduced and levels of gonadotropins are usually elevated. Prolactin level is elevated but the significance is uncertain
Carcinoma of the male breast	Rare tumor. Gynecomastia is unilateral and may be very tender
Medications	
Spironolactone, cimetidine, cyproterone, flutamide	Compete for androgen receptors. Spironolactone also decreases testosterone secretion
Marijuana, digitalis	Weak intrinsic estrogen effects. Marijuana may also compete for androgen receptors
Chemotherapy (alkylating agents)	Predominant effect is on germinal epithelium, but Leydig's cells may be involved
Estrogens, testosterone, hCG	Testosterone treatment of hypogonadism is initially associated with transient gynecomastia produced by peripheral conversion to estradiol. hCG stimulates estradiol secretion in addition to testosterone secretion
Methyldopa, reserpine tricyclic antidepressants	Unknown mechanisms. Serum prolactin level may be elevated, but significance is uncertain

Common causes of hematuria

I. Extrarenal causes
  A. Genitourinary tract diseases
    Calculi—renal pelvis, ureter, bladder, urethra
    Neoplasms—renal pelvis, ureter, bladder, prostate, urethra
    Infections—bladder, prostate, urethra, epididymis
    Others—drugs (cyclophosphamide), foreign bodies, benign
    prostatic hypertrophy, endometriosis, trauma, strictures,
    vesicoureteral reflux
  B. Unrelated to genitourinary tract
    Coagulopathies
    Anticoagulation

II. Renal Parenchymal Causes
  A. Glomerular diseases
    Mesangial proliferative glomerulonephritis (e.g., IgA nephritis)
    Acute proliferative glomerulonephritis (e.g., poststreptococcal nephritis)
    Glomerulonephritis due to systemic diseases (e.g., lupus)
    Rapidly progressive glomerulonephritis (e.g., Goodpasture syndrome)
    Membranoproliferative glomerulonephritis
    Vascular (e.g., malignant hypertension, vasculitides)
    Familial (e.g., Alport syndrome, thin glomerular basement membrane disease)
    Miscellaneous (e.g., loin pain-hematuria syndrome)
  B. Tubulointerstitial diseases
    Infections (e.g., pyelonephritis, tuberculosis)
    Interstitial nephritis, acute (e.g., drugs) chronic (e.g., analgesic abuse)
    Polycystic kidney disease
    Vascular—renal infarction, cortical necrosis, renal vein thrombosis, malformations
    Neoplasms—renal cell carcinoma
    Others—papillary necrosis, trauma, hypercalciuria, hyperuricosuria

Causes of hemoptysis in adults

Infections
  Chronic bronchitis
  Bronchiectasis
  Lung abscess
  Bacterial pneumonias
  Fungal infections
  Tuberculosis
Neoplasms
  Bronchogenic carcinoma
  Bronchial adenoma
  Carcinoma metastatic to the lung
Cardiovascular disorders
  Mitral stenosis
  Pulmonary infarction
  Congenital heart disease, especially cyanotic heart disease
Pulmonary arteriovenous fistula
Parasitic diseases
Pulmonary-renal diseases (Goodpasture's disease)
Miscellaneous
  Cystic fibrosis
  Broncholith
  Cysts and bullae
  Endometriosis (catamenia)
  Idiopathic (in 10%-15% cases no demonstrable cause is found)
  Malingering and/or Münchausen's syndrome

Causes of androgen-dependent hirsutism

I. Ovarian
   A. Neoplastic
      1. Tumors of gonadal stroma
         a. Sertoli-Leydig tumors (arrhenoblastoma)
         b. Granulosa-theca tumors
         c. Sertoli cell tumor
         d. Lipid cell tumor
         e. Gynandroblastoma
      2. Germ cell tumors
         a. Teratoma
      3. Mixed stroma and germ cell tumors
         a. Gonadoblastoma
   B. Nonneoplastic
      1. Idiopathic hirsutism
      2. Polycystic ovary syndrome
      3. Insulin resistance
II. Adrenal
   A. Neoplastic
      1. Adrenal carcinoma
      2. Virilizing adrenal adenoma
   B. Nonneoplastic
      1. Congenital adrenal hyperplasia
         a. 21-Hydroxylase deficiency
         b. 11-Hydroxylase deficiency
         c. 3-Beta-hydroxysteroid dehydrogenase deficiency
      2. Cushing's disease
III. Iatrogenic or factitious
   A. Androgens
         a. Synthetic androgens
         b. Parenteral testosterone esters
   B. "19-nor" progestins

Causes of hypercalcemia

Primary hyperparathyroidism
Cancer
   Parathyroid hormone-related protein
   Ectopic production of 1,25-dihydroxyvitamin D
   Other factors produced ectopically
   Lytic bone metastases
Nonparathyroid endocrine disorders
   Thyrotoxicosis
   Pheochromocytoma
   Adrenal insufficiency
   Vasoactive intestinal polypeptide hormone–producing tumor
Granulomatous diseases (1,25-dihydroxyvitamin D excess)
   Sarcoidosis
   Tuberculosis
   Histoplasmosis
   Coccidioidomycosis
   Leprosy
Medications
   Thiazide diuretics
   Lithium
   Estrogens and antiestrogens
Milk-alkali syndrome
Vitamin A intoxication
Vitamin D intoxication
Familial hypocalciuric hypercalcemia
Immobilization
Parenteral nutrition
Acute and chronic renal insufficiency

Causes of sustained hyperkalemia

Aldosterone deficiency
    Addison's disease
    Hyporeninemic hypoaldosteronism
    Angiotensin-converting enzyme inhibitor therapy
    Prostaglandin synthetase inhibitors
    Corticosterone methyl oxidase deficiency
    Heparin therapy
Decreased response to aldosterone
    Renal failure
        Acute renal failure
        Advanced chronic renal failure
        Severe prerenal azotemia
    Renal tubular disorders
        Obstructive uropathy
        Sickle cell disease
        Renal transplantation
        Amyloidosis
        Systemic lupus erythematosus
        Tubulointerstitial nephropathies
    Potassium-sparing diuretics
    Pseudohypoaldosteronism
    Gordon's syndrome

Causes of hypermagnesemia

I. Decreased renal excretion
    A. Renal failure—glomerular filtration rate less than 30 ml/min
    B. Hyperparathyroidism
    C. Hypothyroidism
    D. Addison's disease
    E. Lithium intoxication
    F. Familial hypocalciuric hypercalcemia
II. Other causes: usually in association with decrease in glomerular filtration rate
    A. Endogenous loads
        1. Diabetic ketoacidosis
        2. Severe tissue injury—burns
    B. Exogenous loads
        1. Gastrointestinal
            a. Magnesium-containing laxatives and antacids
            b. High-dose vitamin D analogs
        2. Parenteral: management of toxemia of pregnancy

Causes of hyperphosphatemia

I. Renal causes
 A. Renal failure
   1. Acute
   2. Chronic
 B. Increased tubular reabsorption of phosphate
   1. Hypoparathyroidism
   2. Pseudohypoparathyroidism
   3. PTH suppression
   4. Acromegaly
   5. Thyrotoxicosis
   6. Bisphosphonate therapy
   7. Tumoral calcinosis
   8. Sickle cell anemia
II. Gastrointestinal causes
 A. Acute phosphate load
   1. Intravenous therapy
   2. Excess oral intake
 B. Surreptitious abuse of phosphate-containing laxatives
 C. Vitamin D overdose
III. Increased cellular release
 A. Rhabdomyolysis
 B. Tumor lysis syndrome
 C. Malignant hyperthermia
 D. Transfusion of stored blood
 E. Respiratory acidosis
 F. Lactic acidosis (?)

Hyperphosphatemia

Causes of hyperprolactinemia

Physiologic
  Pregnancy and lactation
  Sleep
  Stress
  Exercise
  Chest wall stimulation or trauma
  Coitus
Pathologic
  Hypothalamic
    Inflammation
    Tumor
  Pituitary
    Lactotroph microadenoma or macroadenoma
    Acromegaly
    Stalk section caused by pituitary or parasellar mass
    Empty sella syndrome
  Peripheral
    Hypothyroidism
    Chronic renal failure
Pharmacologic
  Psychotropic agents
    Phenothiazines
    Tricyclic antidepressants
    Opiate alkaloids
  Antiemetics and antihistamines
    Metoclopramide
    Sulpiride
    Cimetidine
  Antihypertensives
    Methyldopa
    Reserpine
  Hormones
    Estrogens
    Thyrotropin-releasing hormone

Modified from Melmed S et al: Ann Intern Med 105:238, 1986.

Causes of pulmonary hypertension

Precapillary pulmonary hypertension
    Primary pulmonary hypertension
    Disorders of ventilation
    Congenital heart disease with pulmonary vascular disease
    Pulmonary embolism
    Schistosomiasis
Passive pulmonary hypertension
    Left ventricular failure
    Mitral valve disease
    Cor triatriatum
    Obstruction of major pulmonary veins
Reactive pulmonary hypertension
    Some patients with mitral valve disease
    Rarely, other causes of pulmonary venous hypertension, including
        pulmonary veno-occlusive disease

Causes of fasting hypoglycemia

Drugs
    Insulin
    Sulfonylureas
    Ethanol
    Salicylates
    Pentamidine
    Quinine
Critical organ failure
    Renal failure
    Hepatic failure
    Cardiac failure
    Sepsis
    Malnutrition
Hormonal deficiencies
    Cortisol
    Growth hormone
    Glucagon plus epinephrine
Extrapancreatic tumors
Endogenous hyperinsulinism
    Pancreatic beta-cell disorders: neoplastic (insulinoma), hyperplas-
        tic, or functional
    Insulin secretagogues (e.g., sulfonylureas)
    Autoimmune hypoglycemias: antibodies to insulin, antibodies to
        insulin receptors
Hypoglycemias of infancy and childhood
    Neonatal hypoglycemias
    Congenital deficiencies of glucogenic enzymes
    Ketotic hypoglycemia of childhood

Causes of hypopituitarism

Congenital or acquired
  Septo-optic dysplasia
  Hypogonadotrophic hypogonadism
  Prader-Willi syndrome
  Laurence-Moon-Biedl syndrome
  Isolated GH deficiency
  Neurosecretory GH deficiency
  Basal encephalocele
Vascular
  Pituitary apoplexy
  Sheehan's syndrome
  Arteritides
  Carotid aneurysm
Inflammatory
  Autoimmune lymphocytic hypophysitis
  Histiocytosis
  Sarcoidosis
  Tuberculosis
  Syphilis
  Mycoses
Physical agents
  Cranial trauma and hemorrhage
  Ionizing radiation
  Stalk section
  Surgery
Infiltrations
  Hemochromatosis
  Metastatic carcinoma (breast and bronchus)
  Amyloidosis
Tumors
  Hypothalamic
    Craniopharyngioma
    Glioma
    Germinoma
    Meningioma (sphenoidal ridge)
    Hamartoma
    Leukemia and lymphoma
  Pituitary
    Functioning macroadenomas
    Nonfunctioning macroadenomas
Idiopathic
  Empty sella
  Diabetes insipidus

Causes of orthostatic hypotension

Functional	Neurogenic (autonomic insufficiency)
Reduction in effective blood volume	Familial dysautonomia
Hemorrhage	Shy-Drager syndrome
Prolonged bed rest	Parkinson's disease
Adrenal insufficiency	Tabes dorsalis
Pregnancy	Syringomyelia
Drugs altering vascular reactivity or	Cerebrovascular disease
nervous system function	Peripheral neuropathy due in diabetes
Antihypertensives	Idiopathic orthostatic hypotension
Adrenergic antagonists	Sympathectomy
Ca^{2+} channel blockers	
Antidepressants	
Alcohol and depressants	

Hypotension, orthostatic

Etiology of infectious disease syndromes in the compromised host

Pattern of involvement	Bacteria	Fungi	Viruses	Parasites
Disseminated disease with skin lesions (vasculitis or abscesses, or both)	*Staphylococcus aureus* *Pseudomonas aeruginosa* *Aeromonas hydrophila* Other gram negative bacteria *Nocardia* *Noncholera vibrios* *Mycobacteria*	*Candida* sp. *Aspergillus* Phycomycetes *Trichosporon* sp.	Herpes simplex Varicella-zoster	
Diffuse interstitial pneumonia*	Any gram-negative or gram-positive, including *Nocardia* and mycobacteria	*Aspergillus* *Candida* *Mucor* sp. *Cryptococcus*	Herpes simplex Varicella-zoster Cytomegalovirus Measles	*Pneumocystis carinii* *Toxoplasma gondii* *Strongyloides stercoralis* *T. gondii*
Central nervous system infection, meningoencephalitis, possibly brain abscess	*Listeria monocytogenes* *Nocardia* *S. aureus* *P. aeruginosa* *Mycobacterium tuberculosis*	*Cryptococcus neoformans* *Aspergillus fumigatus* Phycomycetes *Candida* sp.	Varicella-zoster	*T. gondii*
Oroesophageal syndromes	Anaerobes Aerobes: streptococci and gram-negative rods, particularly *P. aeruginosa*	*Candida* *Aspergillus*	Herpes simplex Cytomegalovirus	

Diarrhea	*Clostridium difficile*	Adenovirus	*Giardia lamblia*
	Campylobacter	Coxsackievirus	*Cryptosporidium*
	Salmonella	Rotavirus	*Microsporidia*
	Shigella		*Isospora belli*

*Consider also underlying disease, radiation, and drug reactions.

Causes of magnesium deficiency

Redistribution

Insulin administration
Hungry bone syndrome
Catecholamine excess states
(?) Acute respiratory alkalosis
Acute pancreatitis
Miscellaneous
  Excessive lactation and sweating

Gastrointestinal causes

Reduced intake
  Starvation
  Postoperative
Reduced absorption
  Specific magnesium malabsorption
  Generalized malabsorption syndrome
  Extensive bowel resections
  Diffuse bowel disease or injury
  Chronic diarrhea, laxative abuse

Renal causes

Primary tubular disorders
  Primary renal magnesium wasting
  Welt's syndrome
  Bartter's syndrome
  Renal tubular acidosis
  Diuretic phase of acute tubular necrosis
  Postobstructive diuresis
  Post–renal transplantation status
Extrarenal factors that increase magnesuria
  Drug-induced losses
    Diuretics, aminoglycosides, digoxin, *cis*-platinum, and cyclo-
      sporine
  Hormone-induced magnesuria
    Aldosteronism, hypoparathyroidism, hyperthyroidism
  Ion- or nutrient-induced tubular losses
    Hypercalcemia
    Extracellular fluid volume expansion
    Glucose, urea, mannitol diuresis
  Phosphate depletion
  Alcohol ingestion

Complex causes

Alcoholism
Diabetic ketoacidosis

Common causes of mineralocorticoid excess

With hypertension (primary mineralocorticoid excess)
    Produced by aldosterone
        Aldosterone secretion the *primary* lesion
            Aldosterone secreting adenoma
            Idiopathic hyperaldosteronism
            Dexamethasone suppressible hyperaldosteronism
            Adrenocortical carcinoma
        Aldosterone secretion *secondary* to another lesion
            Renal artery stenosis
            Renin secreting tumor
            Malignant hypertension
            Chronic renal disease
    Produced by some other mineralocorticoid
        Adrenal cancer
        11-Beta hydroxylase deficiency
        17-Hydroxylase deficiency
        Liddle's syndrome
        11-Beta hydroxysteroid dehydrogenase deficiency
        Licorice ingestion
With normal blood pressure
    Chronic renal disease
    Hepatic cirrhosis
    Cardiac failure
    Vomiting
    Diuretic abuse
    Laxative abuse
    Familial chloride diarrhea

Causes of monarthritis

Infection*,†,or‡
Crystal-induced†
Trauma†
Hemarthrosis†,‡
Foreign body‡
Pigmented villonodular synovitis‡
Joint neoplasms‡
Aseptic necrosis‡
Osteochondritis dissecans‡
Mechanical internal derangement†,‡
Sarcoidosis‡
Neuropathic (Charcot's) joint†,‡
Onset of polyarthritis†,‡

*The most important diagnosis.
†Acute.
‡Chronic.

Causes of muscle weakness

I. Primary proximal weakness
   A. Muscle
      1. Endocrine: hyperthyroidism, hypothyroidism, subacute thyroiditis, hyperparathyroidism, acromegaly, Addison's disease (acute adrenal insufficiency), primary aldosteronism, steroid myopathy (Cushing's syndrome; iatrogenic), and male hypogonadism
      2. Metabolic: diabetes mellitus, insulin-induced hypoglycemia, glycogen storage diseases (acid maltase deficiency, muscle phosphorylase deficiency, muscle phosphofructokinase deficiency), lipid storage disease (carnitine deficiency), and alcoholic myopathy
      3. Muscular dystrophies: limb-girdle, Duchenne's, Becker's
      4. Inflammatory myopathies: polymyositis, dermatomyositis, other collagen vascular diseases including rheumatoid arthritis, sarcoidosis, human immunodeficiency virus
      5. Hypercalcemia, hypophosphatemia, hypokalemia, and hyperkalemia of any cause
      6. Drug induced: colchine, chloroquine, cimetidine, amidarone, beta blockers, D-penicillamine, cyclosporin

Causes of muscle weakness—cont'd

II. A. Neuromuscular junction: myasthenia gravis, Eaton-Lambert, botulism, organophosphate poisoning
   B. Peripheral nerve: diabetic proximal neuropathy, Guillain-Barré syndrome, acute intermittent porphyria, tick paralysis, and arsenic poisoning
   C. Anterior horn cell: poliomyelitis, chronic spinal muscular atrophy

III. Primary distal weakness
   A. Muscle: myotonic dystrophy
   B. Peripheral nerve: beriberi, diphtheria, lead, porphyrins, carcinomatous neuropathy, chronic progressive demyelinating neuropathy, peroneal muscle atrophy (Charcot-Marie-Tooth), Guillain-Barré syndrome, Refsum's disease, compressive lesions (root, plexus, nerve)
   C. Anterior horn cell: poliomyelitis, motor neuron disease

IV. Generalized weakness
   A. Decreased cardiac output (mitral stenosis, tricuspid stenosis, mitral regurgitation)
   B. Acute infectious diseases and chronic infectious diseases such as tuberculosis, brucellosis, and trichinosis
   C. Chronic glomerulonephritis and other causes of uremia, including generalized rhabdomyolysis
   D. Pernicious anemia (and other anemias)
   E. Hepatitis
   F. Neurosyphilis
   G. Psychiatric illnesses such as depression
   H. Multiple sclerosis
   I. Mitochondrial myopathy—genetic, zidovudine
   J. L-tryptophan (eosinophilia-myalgia)

Causes of myelopathy and myelitis

Inflammatory
   Infectious
      Bacterial: spirochetal, tuberculous
      Viral: poliomyelitis; herpes HTLV, HIV, zoster; rabies
      Other: rickettsial, fungal, parasitic
   Noninfectious
      Idiopathic transverse myelitis, multiple sclerosis
Toxic/metabolic
   Arsenic
   Pernicious anemia
   Pellagra
   Diabetes mellitus
   Chronic liver disease
Trauma
   Spinal fracture/dislocation
   Stab/bullet wound
   Herniated nucleus pulposus
Compression
   Spinal neoplasm
   Cervical spondylosis
   Extramedullary hematopoiesis
   Epidural abscess
   Epidural hematoma
Vascular
   Arteriovenous malformation
   Periarteritis nodosa
   Lupus erythematosus
   Dissecting aortic aneurysm
Physical agents
   Electrical injury
   Irradiation
Neoplastic
   Spinal cord tumors
   Paraneoplastic myelopathy

Causes of myocardial ischemia in presence and absence of coronary artery disease

  I. Atherosclerotic obstructive coronary artery disease
 II. Nonatherosclerotic coronary artery disease
    A. Coronary artery spasm
    B. Congenital coronary artery anomalies
       1. Anomalous origin of coronary artery from pulmonary artery
       2. Aberrant origin of coronary artery from aorta or another coronary artery
       3. Coronary arteriovenous fistula
       4. Coronary artery aneurysm
III. Acquired disorders of coronary arteries
    A. Coronary artery embolism
    B. Dissection
       1. Surgical
       2. During percutaneous coronary angioplasty
       3. Aortic dissection
    C. Extrinsic compression
       1. Tumors
       2. Granulomas
       3. Amyloidosis
    D. Collagen vascular disease
       1. Polyarteritis nodosa
       2. Temporal arteritis
       3. Rheumatoid arthritis
       4. Systemic lupus erythematosus
       5. Scleroderma
    E. Miscellaneous disorders
       1. Irradiation
       2. Trauma
       3. Kawasaki disease
    F. Syphilis
 IV. Hereditary disorders
    A. Pseudoxanthoma elasticum
    B. Gargoylism
    C. Progeria
    D. Homocystinuria
    E. Primary oxaluria
  V. "Functional" causes of myocardial ischemia in absence of anatomic coronary artery disease
    A. Syndrome X
    B. Hypertrophic cardiomyopathy
    C. Dilated cardiomyopathy
    D. Muscle bridge
    E. Hypertensive heart disease
    F. Pulmonary hypertension
    G. Valvular heart disease; aortic stenosis, aortic regurgitation

Acute interstitial nephritis

Drugs
Antibiotics

Beta lactams (especially ampi-
  cillin, penicillin)
Rifampin
Sulfonamides
Vancomycin
Ciprofloxacin
Cotrimoxazole
Erythromycin
Tetracycline

Nonsteroidal
anti-inflammatory drugs

Diuretics
Thiazides
Furosemide
Triamterene
Ethacrynic acid

Miscellaneous
Cimetidine
Phenindione
Phenytoin
Allopurinol
Interferon

Infection
Bacteria
Legionella
Brucella
Diphtheria
Streptococcus

Viruses
Epstein-Barr virus
Cytomegalovirus
Hantavirus

Other
Mycoplasma
Rocky Mountain spotted fever
Toxoplasma

Idiopathic
Anti-tubular basement mem-
  brane disease
Tubulointerstitial nephritis and
  uveitis (TINUsyndrome)
Other

Diseases associated with different types of neuropathy

	AIDP	CIDP	Axonal SMP	MN	MNMP	Plex	Small
Metabolic							
Diabetes			+	+	+	+	+
Acromegaly*		+	+	+ (CTS)			
Hypothyroidism*			+	+ (CTS)			
Infectious							
AIDS*	+	+	+		+		
Leprosy			+		+		
Connective tissue SLE*	+		+	+	+		
Rheumatoid arthritis			+		+		
Sjögren's syndrome			+		+		
Periarteritis nodosa*			+		+		
Wegener's granulomatosis*			+		+		
Cranial arteritis*			+		+		
Churg-Strauss syndrome			+		+		
Cryoglobulinemia			+		+		
Hypersensitivity angiitis			+		+		
Lyme disease	+		+	+	+		
Idiopathic							
Sarcoidosis*			+		+		

AIDP, acute inflammatory demyelinating polyneuropathy; CIDP, chronic idiopathic demyelinating polyradiculoneuropathy; axonal SMP, axonal sensorimotor polyneuropathy; MN, mononeuropathy; MNMP, mononeuropathy multiplex; plex, plexopathy; small, small-fiber polyneuropathy; CTS, carpal tunnel syndrome; AIDS, acquired immune deficiency syndrome; SLE, systemic lupus erythematosus.

*Central nervous system manifestations may be present.

Acute pancreatitis

Common causes	Occasional causes	Rare causes
Biliary tract disease	Hyperlipemia	Pancreatic cancer
Alcoholism	Surgery	Cystic fibrosis
Idiopathic	Abdominal trauma	Ischemia
	ERCP*	Vasculitis
	Drugs (e.g., azathioprine)	Hereditary pancreatitis
	Infection	
	Peptic ulcer disease	
	Hypercalcemia	
	Renal transplantation	

*Endoscopic retrograde cholangiopancreatography.

Causes of pancytopenia

1. Pancytopenia with hypocellular bone marrow
   a. Acquired aplastic anemia
   b. Constitutional aplastic anemia
   c. Exposure to chemical or physical agents including ionizing irradiation and chemotherapeutic agents
   d. Some hematologic malignancies including myelodysplasia and aleukemic leukemia.
2. Pancytopenia with normal or increased cellularity of hematopoietic origin
   a. Some hematologic malignancies, including myelodysplasia, and some leukemias, lymphomas, and myelomas
   b. Paroxysmal nocturnal hemoglobinuria
   c. Hypersplenism
   d. Vitamin B_{12}, folate deficiencies
   e. Overwhelming infection
3. Pancytopenia with bone marrow replacement
   a. Tumor metastatic to marrow
   b. Metabolic storage diseases
   c. Osteopetrosis
   d. Myelofibrosis

Causes of pericardial disease

Idiopathic disease
Connective tissue disease
    Rheumatoid arthritis
    Rheumatic fever
    Scleroderma
    Lupus erythematosus
Neoplastic disease
    Bronchogenic carcinoma
    Breast cancer
    Lymphoma
    Primary pericardial disease
Infectious disease
    AIDS
    Viral pericarditis
    Tuberculous pericarditis
    Histoplasmosis and other fungal diseases
    Acute pyogenic pericarditis, especially in children
        Haemophilus influenzae
        Neisseria meningitidis
    Infectious endocarditis
    Reiter's syndrome
    Protozoal pericarditis

Causes of pericardial disease—cont'd

Trauma
  Sharp or blunt trauma
  Iatrogenic trauma
  Radiation
Metabolic disease
  Hemodialysis
  Uremia
  Myxedema
  Chylopericardium
  Cholesterol pericarditis
Amyloidosis
Drug-induced and immune reaction disease
  Procainamide
  Hydralazine
  Anticoagulant
  Nicotinic acid
  Postpericardiotomy syndrome
Myocardial infarction
  Acute myocardial infarction
  Dressler's syndrome
Rupture
  Cardiac rupture
  Ruptured aorta
  Aneurysm of the ascending aorta
  Dissecting hematoma

Causes of polyarthritis: inflammatory joint diseases

	Course			Distribution	
Cause	Acute	Intermittent	Chronic	Symmetric	Asymmetric
Rheumatoid arthritis*		±	+	+	±
Systemic lupus erythematosus*		±	±	+	
Other connective tissue diseases		±	±	+	
Crystal deposition diseases		±	+	+	±
Neisserial infection	+			±	+
Hepatitis B	+		±	+	
Rubella	+			+	
Lyme arthritis	±	+	±		+
Bacterial endocarditis	+			+	±
Rheumatic fever	+			+	±
Erythema nodosum	+	±		+	±
Sarcoidosis	+	+	±	+	+
Hypersensitivity to serum or drugs	+	±		+	±
Henoch-Schönlein purpura	+			±	+
Relapsing polychondritis	±	+	±	+	+
Juvenile (rheumatoid) polyarthritis	±	±	+	+	+
Hypertrophic pulmonary osteoarthropathy	±		+	+	
Ankylosing spondylitis*		±	+	±	+
Reiter's disease*	±	±	±	±	+
Enteropathic arthropathy*	±	+	±	±	+
Psoriatic arthritis*		±	+	+	+
Reactive arthritis	+	±	±	±	+
Behçet's disease	±	+	±		+
Familial Mediterranean fever	±	+	±		+
Whipple's disease	±	+	±	±	+
Palindromic rheumatism	±	+		±	+

*The most important diagnoses.
+ = most common; ± = less common.

Conditions that may cause secondary Raynaud's phenomenon

A. After trauma
   1. Related to occupation
      a. Pneumatic hammer disease
      b. Occupational occlusive arterial disease of the hand
      c. Occupational acro-osteolysis
      d. Vasospasm of typists and pianists
   2. Following injury or operation
B. Neurologic conditions
   1. Thoracic outlet syndrome
   2. Carpal tunnel syndrome
   3. Other neurologic diseases
C. Occlusive arterial disease
   1. Arteriosclerosis obliterans
   2. Thromboangiitis obliterans
   3. Postembolic or postthrombotic arterial occlusion
D. Miscellaneous conditions
   1. Scleroderma
   2. Lupus erythematosus
   3. Rheumatoid arthritis
   4. Dermatomyositis
   5. Fabry's disease
   6. Paroxysmal hemoglobinuria
   7. Cold agglutinins or cryoglobulinemia
   8. Primary pulmonary hypertension
   9. Myxedema
   10. Associated with certain neoplasms
   11. Associated with hepatitis B antigenemia
   12. Pheochromocytoma
   13. Ergotism
   14. After combination chemotherapy for testicular cancer

Adapted from Spittell JA Jr: Vasospastic disorders: recognition and management. Cardiovasc Clin 10:279, 1980. With permission of F.A. Davis Co.

Common causes of seizure

Metabolic factors, especially
   Hypoglycemia
   Hypoxia
   Hyponatremia
   Hypocalcemia
   Acid-base disturbances
   Organ failure: renal, hepatic
   Drug withdrawal: alcohol, sedatives
   Drug intoxication: aminophylline, lidocaine
Focal cortex lesions, including
   Infarction
   Contusion
   Tumor
   Abscess
   Meningitis
   Encephalitis
Congenital: hereditary or acquired
   Idiopathic
      Grand mal
      Petit mal
   Perinatal injury
   Maldevelopment
   Degenerations

Etiologic factors in shock

I. Inadequate circulating blood volume (hypovolemic shock)
   A. Acute hemorrhage (e.g., trauma, gastrointestinal bleeding, retroperitoneal bleeding, hemoptysis, hemothorax, ruptured aortic aneurysm)
   B. Plasma volume loss
      1. Intestinal obstruction
      2. Peritonitis, pancreatitis, rapid accumulation of ascites
      3. Splanchnic ischemia
      4. Extensive burns or exudative skin disease
      5. Increased capillary permeability (prolonged hypoxia and ischemia, extensive tissue injury, anaphylaxis, sepsis)
   C. Excessive water and electrolyte losses
      1. Inadequate fluid and salt intake
      2. Excessive sweating
      3. Severe vomiting or diarrhea
      4. Excessive urinary losses (diabetes mellitus, diabetes insipidus, nephrotic syndrome, salt-losing nephropathy, postobstructive uropathy, diuretic phase of acute renal failure, excessive diuretic use)
      5. Acute adrenocortical insufficiency

Etiologic factors in shock—cont'd

II. Impairment of cardiac pump function (cardiogenic shock)
   A. Acute myocardial infarction
   B. Acute valvular regurgitation
   C. Cardiac rupture
   D. Severe congestive heart failure from any cause (ischemic, hypertensive, or valvular heart disease; cardiomyopathy; myocarditis)
III. Mechanical obstruction to central blood flow
   A. Obstruction to venous return or left ventricular filling
      1. Vena cava obstruction
      2. Cardiac tamponade
      3. Tension pneumothorax
      4. Prosthetic mitral valve thrombus
      5. Atrial myxoma
   B. Obstruction to left ventricular output
      1. Dissecting aortic aneurysm
      2. Prosthetic aortic valve thrombus
      3. Severe aortic stenosis
IV. Vasomotor and microvascular dysfunction
   A. Loss of vasomotor tone (neurogenic shock)
      1. Deep general anesthesia, spinal anesthesia
      2. Spinal cord or brain damage (vasomotor center)
      3. Drugs (adrenergic- and ganglionic-blocking agents, barbiturate and other drug overdoses)
      4. Anaphylaxis
   B. Microvascular failure
      1. Infection (septic shock)
         a. Gram-negative sepsis
         b. Other severe bacterial infections
      2. Anaphylaxis
      3. Prolonged shock from any cause

Major causes of thrombocytopenia

I. Decreased platelet production
  A. Megakaryocyte hypoplasia
    1. Aplastic anemia
    2. Myelofibrosis
    3. Leukemia
    4. Marrow invasion by metastatic tumor, granulomas
    5. Viral infection
    6. Radiation myelosuppression
    7. Toxic agents, drugs, antineoplastic chemotherapy
  B. Ineffective thrombopoiesis
    1. Vitamin B_{12} deficiency
    2. Folate deficiency
II. Splenic sequestration, hypersplenism
III. Increased platelet destruction
  A. Non-immune-mediated platelet destruction
    1. Disseminated intravascular coagulation (DIC)
    2. Prosthetic intravascular devices
    3. Extracorporeal circulation
    4. Thrombotic thrombocytopenic purpura (TTP)
  B. Immune-mediated platelet destruction
    1. Drug-induced immune thrombocytopenia
    2. Alloimmune thrombocytopenia
      a. Neonatal
      b. Posttransfusion purpura
    3. Autoimmune thrombocytopenia (ITP)
      a. Idiopathic thrombocytopenic purpura
      b. Secondary to rheumatic diseases, infections, lymphoproliferative disorders

Causes of thyrotoxicosis

Common	Uncommon
Graves' disease	Pituitary adenoma
Subacute thyroiditis	Struma ovarii
Silent	Metastatic thyroid cancer
Painful	Embryonal carcinoma of the
Toxic adenoma	testes
Toxic multinodular goiter	Choriocarcinoma
Excessive thyroxine hormone	Hyperemesis gravidarum
replacement	Isolated pituitary resistance to
Iodide (Jod-Basedow)	thyroid hormone

Causes of obstructive uropathy

I. **Intrinsic causes**
  A. **Intraluminal**
    1. *Intratubular deposition of crystals (uric acid, sulfas)*
    2. *Stones*
    3. *Papillary tissue*
    4. *Blood clots*
  B. **Intramural**
    1. *Functional*
      a. Ureter (ureteropelvic or ureterovesical dysfunction)
      b. Bladder (neurogenic): spinal cord defect or trauma, diabetes, multiple sclerosis, Parkinson's disease, cerebrovascular accidents
      c. Bladder neck dysfunction
    2. *Anatomic*
      a. Tumors
      b. Infection-granuloma
      c. Strictures
II. **Extrinsic causes**
  A. **Originating in the reproductive system**
    1. *Prostate: benign hypertrophy or cancer*
    2. *Uterus: pregnancy, tumors, prolapse, endometriosis*
    3. *Ovary: abscess, tumor, cysts*
  B. **Originating in the vascular system**
    1. *Aneurysms (aorta, iliac vessels)*
    2. *Aberrant arteries (ureteropelvic junction)*
    3. *Venous (ovarian veins, retrocaval ureter)*
  C. **Originating in the gastrointestinal tract: Crohn's disease, pancreatitis, appendicitis, tumors**
  D. **Originating in the retroperitoneal space**
    1. *Inflammations*
    2. *Fibrosis*
    3. *Tumor, hematomas*

Causes of weight loss

I. Weight loss with normal to increased food intake associated with unimpaired appetite
   A. Insulin-dependent diabetes mellitus
   B. Thyrotoxicosis
   C. Pheochromocytoma
   D. Carcinoid
   E. Malabsorption and maldigestion
   F. Intestinal parasite infestation
   G. Diencephalic syndrome
   H. Malignancy (uncommon)
   I. Luft's syndrome
II. Weight loss with normal or decreased food intake
   A. Impaired appetite that in some cases may be coupled with an increased caloric requirement
      1. Malignancy
      2. Psychiatric disorders (including anorexia nervosa)
      3. AIDS
      4. Liver disease
      5. Addison's disease
      6. Uremia
      7. Chronic infection
      8. Chronic lung disease
      9. Chronic inflammatory disease
      10. Cardiac cachexia
      11. Diabetic neuropathic cachexia
      12. Hypothalamic tumor (very rare)
   B. Unimpaired appetite but decrease of food intake secondary to other factors
      1. Gastric ulcer
      2. Duodenal ulcer with outlet obstruction
      3. Postgastrectomy syndrome
      4. Regional enteritis
      5. Ulcerative colitis
      6. Food faddism

Differential Diagnosis

Arthritis of the axial skeleton

	Intervertebral disk space narrowing	Vacuum phenomena	Intervertebral disk space calcification	Bone outgrowths	Apophyseal joint erosion	Apophyseal joint ankylosis	Atlantoaxial subluxation
Rheumatoid arthritis	+	−	−	−	+	±	+
Psoriatic arthritis, Reiter's syndrome	±	−	−	Paravertebral ossification	±	±	+
Ankylosing spondylitis	±	−	±	Syndesmophytes	+	+	+
Juvenile rheumatoid arthritis	+	−	±	−	+	+	+
Degenerative disease of the nucleus pulposus	+	+	−	−	−	−	−
Spondylosis deformans	−	−	−	Osteophytes	−	−	−
Diffuse idiopathic skeletal hyperostosis	−	−	±	Flowing anterolateral ossification	−	−	−
Alkaptonuria	+	+	+	Syndesmophytes (rare)	−	−	−
Infection	+	−	−	−	−	−	−

+ = common presentation; ± = uncommon; − = rare or absent.

Differential diagnosis of breast mass

Inflammatory disease
  Acute bacterial mastitis
  Chronic mastitis
  Fat necrosis
Mammary dysplasia (benign breast disease)
  Adenosis
  Cystic disease
  Duct ectasia
Benign tumors
  Fibroadenoma
  Papilloma
Malignant tumors

Differential diagnosis of bronchiectasis

Postpneumonic infection* (tuberculosis; allergic bronchopulmonary
    aspergillosis; other fungal, postviral, or necrotizing bacterial
    causes)
Cystic fibrosis
Immotile cilia syndrome (Kartagener's syndrome)
Young's syndrome
Opsonic defects (immunoglobulin deficiencies causing recurrent
    sinoplumonary infections)
Compensatory (a result of cicatrization of pulmonary parenchyma)
Recurrent gastroesophageal reflux and aspiration
Congenital
  Tracheobronchomegaly
  Williams-Campbell syndrome (short stature, chest deformities,
      bronchomalacia)
Associated with inflammatory bowel disease
Idiopathic
*Most frequently results in cylindric form.

Calcium homeostasis

Disorders of calcium metabolism—use of circulating measurements of calcium, phosphorus, and PTH concentrations

Serum Ca	Serum P	Plasma PTH	Disorder
↑	↑	↓ or Nl	Increased gut absorption of calcium (vitamin D intoxication, sarcoidosis, milk-alkali syndrome)
↑	↑	↑	Hypercalcemia of any cause and renal failure
↑	↓	↑	Primary hyperparathyroidism
↑	↓	↓ or Nl	Humoral hypercalcemia of malignancy
↓	↓	↑	Vitamin D deficiency, hypomagnesemia*
↓	↑	↑	Pseudohypoparathyroidism, renal failure, acute pancreatitis
↓	↑	Nl or ↓	Primary hypoparathyroidism

*PTH release is stimulated by acute hypomagnesemia. In contrast, chronic hypomagnesemia is associated with low serum PTH. Nl, normal.

Differential features of the cardiomyopathies

Feature	Dilated or congestive	Hypertrophic	Restrictive
Symptoms	Dyspnea, fatigue, orthopnea, cough, leg edema, ascites	Dyspnea, angina, dizziness, syncope, palpitations	Dyspnea, fatigue, leg edema, ascites
Physical findings	Moderate to severe cardiomegaly, sustained apical impulse, S_3 and S_4 common, murmur of mitral or tricuspid regurgitation	Mild cardiomegaly, sustained or bifid apical impulse with prominent atrial impulse, brisk carotid upstroke, S_4 common; ejection systolic murmur along left sternal edge, longer apical systolic murmur, both often increased during Valsalva strain	Mild to moderate cardiomegaly, prominent S_3, mitral or tricuspid regurgitation common, inspiratory increase in venous pressure
Electrocardiogram	Sinus tachycardia, ventricular and atrial enlargement, arrhythmia, bundle branch block	Left ventricular hypertrophy, short P-R, abnormal Q waves, arrhythmias	Low voltage, interventricular and AV conduction defects
Echocardiogram	Dilated cavities, normal wall thicknesses, decreased fractional shortening, evidence of reduced ejection fraction, MR and TR	Normal or small left ventricular cavity, asymmetrical hypertrophy, systolic anterior motion, small left ventricular outflow, characteristic Doppler velocity profile of LVOT obstruction	Normal to mild dilatation of cavity, reduced systolic function, thick walls, pericardial effusion, mitral inflow patterns of LV diastolic dysfunction

Continued.

Differential features of the cardiomyopathies—cont'd

Feature	Dilated or congestive	Hypertrophic	Restrictive
Medical treatment			
Digitalis	Yes	No	Perhaps
Diuretics	Yes	Perhaps	Yes
Vasodilators	Yes	No	Yes
Sympathomimetic amines	Perhaps	No	Perhaps
Vasoconstrictors	No	Yes	No
Beta blockers	No	Yes	No
Calcium blockers	No	Yes	No
Ace inhibitors	Yes	No	No
Disopyramide	No	Yes	No
Surgical treatment	? Transplantation	Ventriculomyectomy	? Transplantation
Prognosis	Progressive worsening	Generally stable	Rapid worsening
Complications	Heart failure, arrhythmias, systemic or pulmonary embolism	Sudden death, arrhythmias, infective endocarditis, heart failure, systemic embolism	Heart failure, arrhythmias

Modified from Wynne J and Braunwald E: The cardiomyopathies and myocarditides, In Braunwald E, editor: Heart disease, Philadelphia 1980, Saunders.

Differential diagnosis of chest pain

Cardiovascular

Ischemic in origin
   Coronary atherosclerosis
   Aortic stenosis
   Hypertrophic cardiomyopathy
   Severe systemic hypertension
   Severe right ventricular
      hypertension
   Aortic regurgitation
   Severe anemia/hypoxia
Nonischemic in origin
   Aortic dissection
   Pericarditis
   Mitral valve prolapse/
      autonomic dysfunction

Gastrointestinal

Esophageal reflux
Esophageal spasm
Esophageal rupture

Pulmonary

Pulmonary
Pneumothorax
Pneumonia

Neuromuscoloskeletal

Thoracic outlet syndrome
Degenerative joint disease of
   cervical/thoracic spine
Costochondritis (Tietze's syn-
   drome)
Herpes zoster

Psychogenic

Anxiety
Depression
Cardiac psychosis
Self-gain

Differential diagnosis of choreic disorders

Huntington's disease
Acute rheumatic chorea (Sydenham's)
Chorea gravidarum
Systemic lupus erythematosis
Chorea-acanthocytosis
Glutaric acidemia
Methylmalonic aciduria
Familial calcification of the basal ganglia
Acute vascular hemichorea
Senile chorea
Spontaneous oral dyskinesia in the edentulous patient
Drug-induced dyskinesias
   Levodopa, bromocriptine
   Anticholinergics
   Antihistamines
   Oral contraceptives
   Neuroleptics

Congenital disorders of blood coagulation

Coagulation factor	Inheritance	Incidence (per million)	Bleeding symptoms	Abnormal screening tests	Biological half-life of protein (hours)	Treatment
I (fibrinogen)	Autosomal recessive	1	Umbilical bleeding at birth, posttrauma hemorrhage	PT, PTT, TT	100	Cryoprecipitate
II (prothrombin)	Autosomal recessive	1	Similar to hemophilia	PT, PTT	72	FFP, rarely pro-thrombin complex concentrates
V	Autosomal recessive	1	Similar to hemophilia	PT, PTT	24	FFP, possibly platelet concentrates
VII	Autosomal recessive	1	Similar to hemophilia	PT	4-6	Recombinant VIIa
VIII (hemophilia)	Sex-linked recessive	100 (milder disease is much more common)	Hemarthrosis, hema-toma, bruising, severe postopera-tive bleeding	PTT	12	VIII concentrates or cryoprecipitate
vWf (von Wille-brand's factor)	Autosomal dominant or recessive	Probably as frequent as hemophilia A	Epistaxis, gingival bleeding, bruising, menorrhagia, se-vere postoperative bleeding	PTT	4-6, for correction of bleeding time	Cryoprecipitate, DDAVP

Factor	Inheritance		Clinical features	Lab test		Treatment
IX (hemophilia B)	Sex-linked recessive	20	Identical to hemophilia	PT, PTT	24	Prothrombin complex concentrates
X	Autosomal recessive	1	Similar to hemophilia	PT, PTT	50	FFP, rarely prothrombin complex concentrates
XI	Autosomal recessive	1	Mild; however, severe postoperative hemorrhage can occur	PTT	60	FFP, level of 25% adequate for hemostasis
XII	Autosomal recessive	1	None	PTT	60	None
XIII	Autosomal recessive	1	Umbilical bleeding at birth, posttrauma hemorrhage, poor wound healing	—	120	FFP monthly, since level of 2% is adequate for hemostasis
Alpha$_2$ antiplasmin	Autosomal recessive	Unknown	Similar to hemophilia	—	Unknown	FFP
Plasminogen activator inhibitor (PAI-1)	Unknown	Unknown	Severe postoperative and posttrauma bleeding	—	Unknown	EACA
Passovoy	Autosomal dominant	Unknown	Similar to factor XI	PTT	Unknown	FFP

FFP, Fresh-frozen plasma; PT, prothrombin time; PTT, partial thromboplastin time; TT, thrombin (clotting) time; DDAVP, 1-deamino-8-D-arginine vasopressin; EACA, epsilon aminocaproic acid.

Neurologic manifestations of the collagen vascular diseases

Entity	Prevalence rate	Genetics	Age of onset	M:F
Systemic lupus erythematosus (SLE)	Rare in general population, CNS complications in 30%-75%	Sporadic	24 mos. after diagnosis	1:9
Temporal arteritis (TA)	Rare	Sporadic	60-80 years of age	M = F
Polymyalgia rheumatica (PMR)	Rare	Sporadic	60-80 years of age	M = F
Granulomatous giant-cell arteritis (GGA) Wegener's (W)	Rare	Sporadic	30-60 years of age (but any age)	M < F
Periarteritis (P)	Rare	Sporadic	30-40 years of age in 50%	M = F
Polymyositis (PM)	$6.3/10^5$	Sporadic	40-70 years of age	5:1
Dermatomyositis (DM)		Sporadic	Child, adult	M = F

CNS, central nervous system; ESR, erythrocyte sedimentation rate; EMG, electromyogram; Ha, headache; CPK, creatine phosphokinase.

Clinical features	Pathology	Therapy
Seizures 54%, CNS 42%, mental change 33%, hemiparesis 12%, paraparesis 4%, movement disorder 4%, polyneuropathy 8%	Microinfarcts in the CNS; globulin in choroid plexus; fibrinoid degeneration	Probably steroids and/or immunosuppressive therapy
Headache (temporal more than occipital), fever, weight loss, ESR >50 mm; prominent temporal artery; 30% can go blind; CNS involved	Giant-cell arteritis in media of vessels	Temporal artery biopsy, steroids for at least 6 mos
Malaise, weight loss, ESR >50 mm; brainstem strokes occasionally; normal enzymes, EMG; not much weakness	Can show similar pathology as TA or nothing	Steroids until ESR remains low
CNS: seizures, hemiparesis, SAH, infarcts, MS change. PNS: mononeuritis multiplex, neuropathy	Granulomatous lesions in resp. tract, kidneys; vasculitis in nerves and CNS	Steroids and/or immunosuppressives (especially cyclophosphamide)
Acute or insidious; fever, malaise, weakness, arthralgias, visceral involvement. PNS: neuropathies 50%. CNS: Sz, HA, psychosis	Inflammatory arteritis of medium-sized arteries, vasonervorum ischemia; progressive	Steroids
Subacute girdle muscle weakness 98%; dysphagia 51%; muscle pain 58%; ESR, CPK, EMG abnormalities in the majority	?sensitized lymphocytes; ?virus; Degenerative and inflammatory changes in muscle with perivascular lymphs and plasma cells	Steroids; for severe, relapsing cases immunosuppressives may be of benefit
Skin findings in DM; often associated with cancer	Skin DM involved	

SAH,subarachnoid hemorrhage; MS, mental status; PNS, peripheral nervous system; Sz, seizure;

Differential diagnosis of dysuria

   I. Urinary tract infection
      A. Enterobacteriaceae
      B. Gram-positive organisms
      C. *Chlamydia trachomatis*
      D. *Mycobacterium tuberculosis*
  II. Vaginitis
      A. Fungi *(Candida albicans)*
      B. Bacterial
         1. *Gardnerella vaginalis (Haemophilus vaginalis)*
         2. *Neisseria gonorrhoeae*
         3. *Treponema pallidum* (endourethral chancre)
         4. *Chlamydia trachomatis*
      C. Protozoa *(Trichomonas vaginalis)*
 III. Genital infection
      A. Herpes simplex (genitalis)
      B. Condyloma accuminatum
      C. Paraurethral glands
  IV. Estrogen deficiency
   V. Interstitial cystitis (Hunner's ulcer)
  VI. Reiter's syndrome
 VII. Chemical irritants
      A. Douches
      B. Deodorant aerosols
      C. Contraceptive jellies
      D. Bubble bath
VIII. Impedance to flow
      A. Urethral caruncle or diverticula
      B. Meatal stenosis or stricture
      C. Transient urethral edema
      D. Chronic fibrosis after trauma
      E. Impaired synergy: bladder contraction and sphincter relaxation
  IX. Regional disease
      A. Crohn's disease
      B. Diverticulitis
      C. Cervical radium implant
   X. Bladder tumor

Differential diagnosis of epilepsy

Disorder	Unlike epilepsy	Like epilepsy
Syncope	Premonitory symptoms Precipitating factors Diffuse fading vision	Myoclonic jerks or tonic stiffening, on occasion
Transient ischemic attack	No "march" of symptoms No jerks, twitches No loss of consciousness, amnesia Brainstem symptoms	Focal EEG slowing Normal examination between attacks
Migraine	Prominent headache Preserved consciousness	Focal symptoms Focal EEG slowing
Hypoglycemia	Temporal relationship to fasting Initial sympathetic discharge	Focal symptoms and EEG slowing Loss of consciousness Postictal headache, confusion
Paroxysmal vertigo	Preserved consciousness Monosymptomatic spells Auditory, vestibular abnormalities	Severe temporary disability
Narcolepsy	Cataplexy Appropriate sleep behavior with attacks	Hallucinations
Psychogenic spells	Event-related Stressful context Lack of autonomic features Lack of incontinence	Inappropriate, unpredictable timing of attacks Dramatic convulsive behavior

Facial pain

	Location	Nature	Timing	Associated physical findings
Tic douloureux	V2, then V2-V3; rarely V1	Triggered	Brief jabs	None
Geniculate neuralgia	Ear	Not often triggered	Brief jabs, or long duration	Vesicles in ear, VII palsy, ± VIII findings
Glossopharyngeal neuralgia	Tonsillar fossa, ear	Triggered	Brief jabs	Episodes of syncope
Postherpetic neuralgia	One or more adjacent cranial or cervical nerves	Burning	Constant	Healed skin lesions, sensory loss, or hyperpathia
Posttraumatic neuralgia	Usually one cranial or cervical nerve	Burning, aching	Constant	Sensory disturbances
Cluster headache	Retro-orbital, cheek, temple	Boring, deep, intense	Attacks of 30-120 min	Lacrimation, ptosis, rhinorrhea
"Lower-half headache"	Orbit, nose, cheek, mastoid; may spread to neck and arm	Boring, deep, intense	Attacks lasting one or more hours	Sometimes flushing, lacrimation, rhinorrhea
Carotidynia	One side of neck	Deep, aching	Several days	Tender carotid in neck
Atypical facial pain	Cheek, jaw, entire face	Aching, may be bizarre	Constant	Emotional disturbance

Identification of life-threatening diseases associated with fever and rash

Disease	History	Characteristics of rash	Distribution of rash	Associated clinical findings	Diagnostic aids
Rocky Mountain spotted fever	Tick exposure (75%) May-September occurrence in temperate-zone states Heaviest endemic area middle Atlantic states and Southeast	Initial maculopapular petechiae appearing on 2nd to 6th febrile day and usually painless	Begins on wrists, ankles, forearms, spreading within 6-8 hours to palms, soles, trunk	Prodrome of fever, headache, myalgias Hyponatremia, normal to slightly increased WBC, thrombocytopenia, hypoalbuminemia	Biopsy of involved skin with immunofluorescence and other serologic tests Serology: Complement-fixation more sensitive and more specific than Weil-Felix agglutination
Meningococcemia*	Tends to occur in late winter, early spring Outbreaks in military recruits, crowded living conditions	*Acute:* May be maculopapular initially. Small petechiae with irregular borders ("smudging"), at times with vesicular or grayish ulcer. May coalesce. Painful	*Acute:* Extremities and, trunk in random fashion	*Acute:* Meningitis, disseminated intravascular coagulation, shock, acidosis	*Acute:* Aspiration of center of skin lesions for Gram stain, culture (up to 60% positive). Blood cultures. Cerebrospinal fluid culture and Gram stain
		Chronic: Maculopapules, petechial vesicles, or pustules; tender nodules	*Chronic:* Extremities, particularly over joints	*Chronic:* Rash appears with recurrent cycles of fever over 2-3 months	*Chronic:* Blood culture usually positive during febrile episode. Biopsy findings resemble leukocytoclastic angiitis

Continued.

Identification of life-threatening diseases associated with fever and rash—cont'd

Disease	History	Characteristics of rash	Distribution of rash	Associated clinical findings	Diagnostic aids
Disseminated gonococcal infection	Incidence higher in women than in men. Young, sexually active. Onset often related to menstruation	Pustules on erythematous base most characteristic. Also, macules, papules, pustules, and bullae less commonly	Over extremities, with relative sparing of face and trunk. Usually few (5-40) lesions	Migratory polyarthralgia, tenosynovitis, septic arthritis	Gram stain of lesion. Blood, joint fluid culture (50%) prove diagnosis. Cervical, rectal, throat cultures support diagnosis
Staphylococcal septicemia	Nosocomial: indwelling catheters, pacemakers, dialysis shunts, wound infections. Drug abuse	Pustules, purulent purpura, subcutaneous nodules, infarcts	Widespread, with infarcts having predilection for distal extremities	Endocarditis, with valvular incompetence, meningitis, multiple-organ involvement	Aspiration of lesions for Gram stain culture. Blood, cerebrospinal fluid (where indicated) cultures. Teichoic acid antibody suggestive of deep-seated infection

Pseudomonas septicemia	Hospitalized patients, especially with neutropenia or burns	*Vesicles:* Isolated or in small clusters rapidly becoming hemorrhagic	Random	Generally extremely toxic, with fever; septic picture	Aspiration of lesion for Gram stain, culture
		Ecthyma gangrenosum: Round, indurated, ulcerated painless lesion with central gray eschar	Axillary or anogenital area, thigh		Cultures of blood, urine, sputum, etc.
		Maculopapular lesion: Small erythematous lesion resembling "rose spots"	Trunk		
		Gangrenous cellulitis	Localized		
Candida septicemia	Broad-spectrum antibiotics, leukemia, immunosuppression, hyperalimentation, cardiac surgery	Multiple discrete pink maculopapular lesions 2-5 mm in diameter	Trunk and extremities	Toxic state; associated ophthalmitis, esophagitis, cystitis	Punch biopsy of lesion with stains for fungus
					Buffy coat of blood
					Blood cultures (definitive diagnosis)
					Examination and culture of stool, urine, sputum (supportive of diagnosis with multiple-site involvement)
					Barium or endoscopic examination of esophagus

Continued.

Identification of life-threatening diseases associated with fever and rash—cont'd

Disease	History	Characteristics of rash	Distribution of rash	Associated clinical findings	Diagnostic aids
Infective endocarditis	Indwelling catheters, pacemakers, dialysis shunts, valvular heart disease, prosthetic valves, intravenous drug abuse, preceding dental or surgical manipulations	*Petechiae:* often in small groups *Osler's nodes:* pea-sized, tender, erythematous nodules *Janeway's lesions:* small erythematous or hemorrhagic macules	Conjunctivae, palate, upper chest, distal extremities Pads of fingers and toes Palms and soles	Heart murmur, valvular incompetence, metastatic abscesses, infarcts, Roth's spots, splenomegaly, hematuria, glomerulonephritis, etc.	Serology not yet reliable Blood cultures (3-5 sets) Echocardiogram Circulating immune complexes
Toxic shock syndrome	Young female predominance 1-4 days prodrome of fever, myalgias, arthralgias, and diarrhea Onset during or soon after menses (has also been reported in men and unassociated with menses in women)	*Erythroderma:* Seen at presentation. Diffuse, blanching, macular (deep-red "sun-burned" appearance). Resolves within 3 days, followed 5-12 days later by desquamation, most commonly of hands and feet *Mucosal hyperemia:* pharynx, conjunctivae, vagina	Diffuse, hands and feet predominantly	Fever, severe hypotension, multisystem involvement (gastrointestinal, muscular, renal, hepatic, hematologic, central nervous system)	Clinical criteria Negative serology for RMSF, leptospirosis, measles Identification of toxin-producing strain of *S. aureus*

Gastrointestinal infections, AIDS patients

| Lyme disease | From endemic areas—Northeast, Midwest (Minnesota/Wisconsin), and West (California/Oregon) Usually begins in summer | *Erythema chronicum migrans*: Expanding annular erythema (median diameter 15 cm) from central macule or papule. Secondary annular lesions seen | Commonly thigh, groin, axilla. Any site can be involved | Fever, chills, malaise, myalgias, lymphadenopathy Late (weeks to months) central nervous system, cardiac, and joint involvement | Primarily history and clinical criteria Organism can be cultured (difficult, special media) Serology |

*Acute syndrome may occasionally be caused by *Haemophilus influenzae* and *Streptococcus pneumoniae*, especially in splenectomized patients.

Gastrointestinal infections commonly associated with AIDS and the pathogens frequently causing these infections

Proctitis

Herpes simplex virus
Neisseria gonorrhoeae
Treponema pallidum
Chlamydia trachomatis

Colitis

Salmonella species
Campylobacter species
Shigella species
Entamoeba histolytica
Cytomegalovirus

Enteritis

Cryptosporidium
Isospora belli
Giardia lamblia
Strongyloides stercoralis
Mycobacterium avium-intracellulare
Cytomegalovirus

Differential diagnosis of genital lesions

Morphology	Number	Distribution	Surface	Base
Ulcers	?Single (55%) or multiple	Penis, labia, cervix	Clean	Indolent
	Single	Penis	Purulent	Inflamed
	Single	Penis, labia	Beefy red, granulation tissue	Friable
	Single	Penis, labia	Eroded papule	Benign
	Multiple	Penis, vulva, thigh, cervix, grouped	Clean	Clean, all same size
	Multiple (30%) or single (70%)	Penis, vulva, thigh	Necrotic	Variable size, ragged
Papules	Single	Penis, labia	Clean or small erosion	Benign
	Multiple	One or more rows behind corona	Clean	Benign
	Multiple	Penis, labia, vagina, often grouped	Verrucous	Benign
	Multiple	Penis, labia, pubic hair, thighs, buttocks	Umbilicated, with tiny plug	Benign
	Multiple	Disseminated, palms, soles	Coppery	Benign
	Multiple	Penis, labia, thighs, buttocks, wrists, and ankles	Crusted	
Vesicles	Multiple	Penis, labia, thighs, cervix, grouped	Umbilicated	Erythema
Crusts	Multiple	Grouped		Erythema
	Multiple	Disseminated		Erythema may be present
Erythema	Patches	Glans, shaft of penis, labia, vulva	Intense erythema	

Edge	Pain	Adenopathy	Incubation period	Suggested diagnosis
Indurated	Mild (30%)	Moderate	<21 d (up to 90 d)	Syphilis
Ragged	Mild to severe	Mild or absent	<24 h	Human bite, other trauma
Serpiginous		Inguinal granulomas	1-12 wk	Donovanosis
Benign	Lesion often goes entirely unnoticed	Moderate, but usually appears after lesion resolves	2 wk	Lymphogranuloma venereum
Erythema	Severe: prodome of paresthesia	Moderate, tender	3-7 d, recurrent	Herpes genitalis
Undermined erythema	Moderate	Moderate, tender	2-5 d	Chancroid
Benign			2 wk	Early lymphogranuloma venereum
Benign				Pearly penile papules
Benign			3-30 wk	Venereal warts
Benign			2-26 wk	Molluscum contagiosum
Benign	Occasional, mild	Prominent	6-12 wk	Secondary syphilis
Linear tracks may be seen	Intense pruritus	Rare superinfected excoriation	4 wk	Scabies
	Mild	Moderate, tender	2-5 d	Herpes genitalis
	Mild	Mild	2-5 d	Healing herpes genitalis
	Pruritus	Mild or absent	4 wk	Scabies
Satellite lesions	Pruritus		Undefined	Candidiasis

Summary of primary renal diseases that normally present as acute glomerulonephritis

Diseases	Poststreptococcal glomerulonephritis	IgA nephropathy	Goodpasture's syndrome	Idiopathic crescentic nephritis
Clinical manifestations				
Age and sex	All ages, mean 7, 2:1 male	15-35, 2:1 male	15-30, 6:1 male	Mean 58, 2:1 male
Acute nephritic syndrome	90%	50%	90%	90%
Asymptomatic hematuria	Occasionally	50%	Rare	Rare
Nephrotic syndrome	10-20%	Rare	Rare	10-20%
Hypertension	70%	30-50%	Rare	25%
Acute renal failure*	50% (transient)	Very rare	50%	60%
Other	1-3 week latent period	Follows viral syndromes	Pulmonary hemorrhage Iron-deficiency anemia	None
Recurs in transplants	No	Yes	Only if antibody present	No
Laboratory findings	ASO titers (70%) Positive streptozyme (95%) C3-C9, normal C1, C4	Increased IgA-fibronectin aggregates IgA in dermal capillaries	Positive anti-GBM antibody	Increased anti-neutrophil cytoplasmic antibody (ANCA)

Immunogenetics	HLA D "EN" (9)* ? DR4 (4)	DR4 (4), ? HLA Bw 35	HLA DR2 (16), B7 (5)	None established
Renal pathology				
Light microscopy	Diffuse proliferation	Focal proliferation	Focal diffuse proliferation with crescents	Crescentic GN
Immunofluorescence	Granular IgG, C3	Diffuse mesangial IgA, IgG	Linear IgG, C3	No immune deposits
Electron microscopy	Subepithelial humps	Mesangial deposits	No deposits	No deposits
Treatment	Supportive	None established	Plasma exchange, steroids cyclophosphamide	Steroid pulse therapy, cyclophosphamide
Prognosis	95% resolve spontaneously 5% RPGN or slowly progressive	Slow progression in 25%-50%	75% stabilize or improve if treated early	75% stabilize or improve if treated early

*Relative risk.
RPGN, rapidly progressive glomerulonephritis.

Differential diagnosis of granulomatous lung disease

Infections

Bacteria
  Brucella
  Francisella tularensis
  Yersinia enterocolitica
Mycobacteria
  Tuberculosis
  Atypical tuberculosis
Fungi
  Histoplasma capsulatum
  Blastomyces dermatitidis
  Coccidioides immitis
Spirochetes: *Treponema*

Nonfectious compounds

Organic: hypersensitivity pneumonitis
Inorganic
  Beryllium
  Talc
Drugs
  Methotrexate
  Dilantin
Neoplasms
  Lymphoma
  Germ cell cancer

Idiopathic

Sarcoidosis
Wegener's granulomatosis
Primary biliary cirrhosis
Crohn's disease
Ulcerative colitis

Important headache syndromes

Incidence	Age of onset	Sex bias	Family history of headaches	Onset and evolution of headache	Time course of headache	Quality	Location	Exacerbators	Associated features	Physical signs
Migraine										
Without aura										
Common	Childhood, adolescence, or young adulthood	Female	Yes	Slow to rapid	Episodic	Usually throbbing	Variable, often unilateral	Head-low position, exertion	Prodrome, vomiting	No
With aura										
Uncommon	Childhood, adolescence, or young adulthood	Female	Yes	Slow to rapid	Episodic	Usually throbbing	Variable, generally unilateral	Head-low position, exertion	Prodrome, aura, vomiting	No
Cluster headache										
Uncommon	Young adulthood, middle age	Male	No	Rapid	Clusters in time	Constant	Orbit, temple cheek	None	Lacrimation, rhinorrhea, Horner's syndrome	Partial Horner's syndrome
Tension-type headache										
Very common	Young adulthood, middle age	No	Yes	Slow to rapid	Episodic, may become constant	Constant	Variable	Stress	None	No

Temporal arteritis Uncommon	Over 50	No	Slow	Increasing, becoming constant	Constant	Localized	None	Generally ill	Arterial changes, fever
Subarachnoid hemorrhage Uncommon	Over 35	No	Abrupt	Persists for days	Constant	Diffuse	None	Altered consciousness, sometimes vomiting	Meningeal irritation, sometimes focal signs
Meningitis Uncommon	Any age	No	Rapid	Persists for days	Constant	Diffuse	None	Altered consciousness, sometimes vomiting	Meningeal irritation, sometimes focal signs
Brain tumor Uncommon	Any age	No	Slow	Duration steadily increases	Constant, localized, then diffuse	Localized, then diffuse	Head-low position, exertion	Altered consciousness, sometimes vomiting	Focal signs common, sometimes papilledema

The ABCs of viral hepatitis

	Hepatitis A	Hepatitis B
Incubation period	2-6 wks	2-6 months
Onset	Usually acute	Usually insidious
Symptoms		
Nausea and vomiting	Common	Common
Fever	Common	Uncommon
Jaundice	50%	33%
Arthralgias	Rare	Common
Diagnosis	IgM Anti-HAV	HBsAg
Transmission		
Fecal-oral	Usual	Rare (not fecal)
Parenteral	Rare	Usual
Sexual	Yes	Yes
Perinatal	No	Yes
Sequelae		
Chronic carrier	No	5%-10%
Chronic active hepatitis	No	Approximately 5%
Fulminant hepatitis	Approximately 0.1%	0.2%-1.0%
Recovery	Greater than 99%	85%-90%
Epidemiology		
Sporadic cases	Mainly children in developing countries and adults in developed countries	Primarily males
Epidemics	Foodborne or waterborne	Contaminated blood products (vaccines, dialysis machines, IV drug users)
Post-transfusion	Extremely rare	Less than 5% of post-transfusion cases
Prevention	ISG†	HBIG†, vaccine

*10%-20% fatalities in pregnant women.
†*ISG,* human immune serum globulin; *HBIG,* hepatitis B immune globulin.

Hepatitis C	Hepatitis D	Hepatitis E
2-22 wks	4-8 wks	2-9 wks
Usually insidious	Usually acute	Usually acute
Common	Common	Common
Uncommon	Uncommon	Uncommon
25%	?	10%-20%
Rare	Rare	Rare
Anti-HCV	IgM anti-HDV	Anti-HEV
Rare	?	Usual
Usual	Usual	No
?Rare	?	?
?Rare	?	No
Up to 60%	?Most	No
?30%-50%	Up to 70%	No
?	Up to 17%	2%-10%*
?	?	90%-98%*
40%-50% of sporadic hepatitis cases	—	Young to middle-aged adults
Contaminated blood products	Contaminated blood products, IV drug users	Foodborne or waterborne
85%-95% of post-transfusion cases	Possible	No
? ISG†	Hepatitis B vaccine	?ISG† from endemic areas

Differential diagnosis of hyperinsulinism

	Postabsorptive venous plasma glucose <45 mg/dl			
	Insulin	C peptide	Insulin antibodies	Other
Exogenous hyperinsulinism	↑	↓†	+	
Endogenous hyperinsulinism				
Insulinoma	↑	↑	—	↑ Proinsulin
Sulfonylurea	↑	↑	—	Positive sulfonylurea assay
Autoimmune hypoglycemia				
Antibodies to insulin	↑↑↑*	↓†	+	
Antibodies to insulin receptor	↑	?	—	Insulin receptor antibodies present; associated autoimmune disorder

*Insulin antibodies artifactually increase insulin levels measured by double-antibody radioimmunoassay.

†Free C-peptide levels are low, but total C-peptide levels may not be because of cross reactivity with antibody-bound proinsulin.

Differential diagnosis of hypocalcemia

Situational
    Hypoalbuminemia
    Alkalosis
    Elevated concentrations of free fatty acids
    Intensive care unit–associated
Hypoparathyroidism
    Postsurgical hypoparathyroidism
    Idiopathic hypoparathyroidism
        Isolated
        Multiple glandular failure
    Magnesium deficiency, severe
    Hypermagnesemia
    Infiltrative diseases of parathyroid glands
        Hemochromatosis
        Thalassemia
        Wilson's disease
        Metastatic carcinoma
        Amyloidosis
    Ionizing radiation or chemotherapy
    Congenital disorders (DiGeorge's syndrome, Kearns-Sayre syndrome)
    Neonatal hypocalcemia
Relative hypoparathyroidism
    Acute pancreatitis
    Acute release of cellular phosphate
        Rhabdomyolysis
        Chemotherapy
        Toxic shock syndrome
    Osteoblastic metastases
    Multiple, citrated blood transfusions
    States of 1,25-dihydroxyvitamin D deficiency
    Some vitamin D resistant states
Resistance to parathyroid hormone
    Pseudohypoparathyroidism
        Type Ia and type Ib
        Type II
        Split target organ sensitivity

Clinical and radiologic differentiation of ulcerative colitis and Crohn's colitis

Findings	Ulcerative colitis	Crohn's colitis
Clinical findings		
Hematochezia	Present in most patients	Present in 50% of patients
Abdominal pain	Mild, rarely severe	Severe in 50% of patients
Abdominal mass	None	Present in 10% of patients
Perianal lesions	Present in 20% of patients, rarely severe	Present in 80% of patients, often severe
Proctosigmoidoscopic findings	Distal involvement in virtually all patients	Distal involvement in 50% of patients
	Uniformly granular mucosa	Patchy granularity, cobblestones
		Discrete ulcers with or without normal intervening mucosa

Radiologic findings

Distribution	Rectum involved in most patients	Rectum involved in 50% of patients
	Continuous disease	Often discontinuous disease
Contour	Bowel uniformly contracted and shortened	Bowel of varying diameter and rarely shortened
	Involvement usually concentric	Segmental, eccentric involvement
		Pseudodiverticula
		Incomplete haustral loss
Mucosal detail	Absence of haustral pattern (late in disease)	Irregular, nodular, cobblestone pattern
	Generalized granular outline	Aphthous ulcers
	Loss of folds	Deep, transverse, linear fissures (spiking)
	Diffuse shallow (<2 mm) ulceration, may be deeper	Longitudinal ulceration
		Pseudopolyps less extensive
Small bowel	Pseudopolyps prominent	Thickened ileocecal valve
	Gaping ileocecal valve	Terminal ileum narrowed, irregular
	Terminal ileum may be dilated	Involvement may be discontinuous
	Backwash ileitis in 10% of patients	
Internal fistulas	Vary rare, occasionally into vagina	Common
		Occasional intramural or pericolic abscesses

Differential diagnosis of abnormal lymphocytes in peripheral blood

Lymphocyte type	Usual disease association	Cytologic features	Laboratory features	Clinical features
Small lymphocyte	Chronic lymphocytic leukemia	B cell surface markers with low concentration of surface immunoglobulin, CD5 antigen	Hypogammaglobulinemia in 50%; positive direct Coombs' test in 15%; on node biopsy, diffuse, well-differentiated lymphocytic infiltrate	Elderly adults; presentation runs gamut from asymptomatic with lymphocytosis only to bulky disease with adenopathy, splenomegaly, and "packed" bone marrow
Atypical lymphocyte	Infectious mononucleosis, other viral illnesses	Suppressor T cell markers	Heterophil agglutinin; positive serology for Epstein-Barr virus, cytomegalovirus, toxoplasma, HBsAg	Pharyngitis, fever, adenopathy, rash, splenomegaly, palatal petechiae, jaundice
Plasmacytoid lymphocyte	Waldenström's macroglobulinemia	Cytoplasmic IgM, periodic acid-Schiff (PAS) positivity	IgM paraprotein, rouleaux, cryoglobulins	Adenopathy, splenomegaly, absence of bone lesions, hyperviscosity syndrome, cryopathic phenomena
Lymphoblast	Acute lymphoblastic leukemia (ALL)	Terminal transferase positivity, common ALL antigen	Anemia, granulocytopenia, thrombocytopenia, hyperuricemia, diffuse bone marrow infiltration	Peak incidence in childhood, acute onset, bone pain frequent

Lymphosarcoma cell	Lymphocytic lymphoma	B cell surface markers with high concentration of surface immunoglobulin	Nodular, or diffuse, poorly differentiated lymphocytic lymphoma on node biopsy, patchy, peritrabecular bone marrow involvement	Middle-aged to older adults, generalized adenopathy, constitutional symptoms
Sézary cell	Cutaneous lymphomas	T lymphocyte surface markers	Skin biopsy is diagnostic	Exfoliative erythroderma, cutaneous plaques or tumors
Hairy cell	Hairy cell leukemia	B lymphocyte markers, cytoplasmic projections, tartrate-resistant acid phosphatase, interleukin-2 receptors, CD11 antigen	Pancytopenia	Middle-aged males, moderate to marked splenomegaly without adenopathy
Prolymphocyte	Prolymphocytic leukemia	B cell surface markers with high concentration of surface immunoglobulin	Marked lymphocytosis (frequently $>100 \times 10^9$/L)	Elderly adults, massive splenomegaly, minimum adenopathy, poor response to therapy

Key features and treatment of the major categories of bladder-emptying dysfunction

Dysfunction	Site of lesion	Voiding pattern	Treatment
Detrusor hyperactivity			
Coordinated sphincter	Cerebrum or basal ganglia, dementia, Parkinson's, CVA, multiple sclerosis	Urgency, urge incontinence voiding without awareness	Anticholinergics
External sphincter dyssynergia	Suprasacral spinal cord	Incomplete emptying, low volume, uninhibited contractions	Anticholinergics, intermittent catheterization
Internal sphincter dyssynergia	Cord lesion above T6-T12	Incomplete emptying, autonomic dysreflexia	Phenoxybenzamine, anticholinergics
Detrusor areflexia			
Coordinated sphincter	Sacral cord or cauda equina	Interrupted flow, voiding by straining	Bethanechol, intermittent catheterization, credé
External sphincter overactivity	Sacral cord	Decreased sensation of fullness, voiding by straining	Bethanechol, diazepam, intermittent catheterization
External sphincter denervation	Sacral cord, peripheral nerves, cauda equina	Incontinence, large residual urine	Intermittent catheterization
Poor relaxation of smooth-muscle sphincter	Sacral cord	High capacity	Phenoxybenzamine, bethanechol

Distinguishing features of chronic myeloproliferative disorders

	CML	IMF	PV	ET
Leukocytes	↑ ↑ ↑	↑ /N/ ↓	↑	N/ ↑
Hematocrit	↓	↓	↑ ↑ ↑	N
Platelets	↑ ↑	↑ /N/ ↓	↑ ↑	↑ ↑ ↑
LAP score	↓	↑ /N/ ↓	↑ ↑ ↑	N/ ↑
Teardrop RBC	−	↑ ↑ ↑	−	−
Marrow fibrosis	±	↑ ↑ ↑	−	−
Ph¹ chromosome	+	−	−	−

CML, chronic myelogenous leukemia; IMF, idiopathic myelofibrosis; PV, polycythemia vera; ET, essential thrombocythemia; LAP, leukocyte alkaline phosphatase. ↑ ↑ ↑, marked increase; ↑ ↑, moderate increase; ↑, slight increase; ±, variable; +, present; −, absent; N, normal; ↓, decrease.

Myeloproliferative disorders

Summary of primary renal diseases that present as idiopathic nephrotic syndrome

Diseases	Minimal change disease	Focal glomerular sclerosis	Membranous nephropathy	Membranoproliferative glomerulonephritis	
				Type I	Type II
Frequency*					
Children	75%	10%	<5%		10%
Adults	15%	15%	50%		10%
Clinical manifestations					
Age	2-6, some adults	2-6, some adults	40-50%		5%-15%
Sex	2:1 male	1.3:1 male	2:1 male		2:1 female
Nephrotic syndrome	100%	90%	80%		60%
Asymptomatic proteinuria	0	10%	20%		40%
Hematuria	No	40%	20%		80%
Hypertension	10%	20% early	Infrequent		35%
Rate of progression	Does not progress	10 years	50% in 10-20 years	10-20 years	5-15 years
Associated conditions	Allergy to NSAIDs Hodgkin's disease	Heroin nephropathy AIDS	Renal vein thrombosis, cancer, SLE, hepatitis	None	Partial lipodystrophy
Recurs in transplants	Yes	50%	Rarely	30%	90%

Laboratory findings	Manifestations of nephrotic syndrome	Manifestations of nephrotic syndrome	Manifestations of nephrotic syndrome	Low C1, C4, C3-C9	Normal C1, C4; low C3-C9; C3 nephritic factor
Immunogenetics	DR7 (6)[†]	DR4 (5-6)	DR3 (2-12)	None	DR7 (9)
Renal pathology					
Light microscopy	Normal	Focal sclerotic lesions	Thickened GBM, spikes	Thickened GBM, proliferation, lobulation	Same as type I
Immunofluorescence	Negative	IgM, C3 in sclerotic	Fine granular IgG, C3	Granular IgG, C3	C3 only
Electron microscopy	Foot process fusion	Lesions, foot process fusion	Subepithelial deposits	Mesangial and subendothelial deposits	Dense deposits
Response to steroids	90%	20%-40%, may slow progression	Slows progression	None established	None established
Other treatment	None	None	Steroids and cytotoxic drugs in high risk patients		

*Approximate frequency as a cause of idiopathic nephrotic syndrome. About 10% of adult nephrotic syndrome is due to various diseases that usually present with acute glomerulonephritis
[†]Relative risk
NSAIDs, nonsteroidal anti-inflammatory drugs; SLE, systemic lupus erythematosus.

Types of nystagmus with localizing value and the common location and cause of the responsible lesions

Type of nystagmus	Common location of responsible lesion	Common causes of responsible lesion
Up-beat nystagmus		
Worse on upgaze	Brainstem or cerebellar vermis	Alcoholic cerebellar degeneration
Worse on downgaze	Medulla or pons	Multiple sclerosis, anticonvulsants, neoplasm
Down-beat nystagmus	Cervicomedullary junction	Cranial malformation, multiple sclerosis, infarction, anticonvulsants, alcoholic cerebellar degeneration, lithium toxicity
Periodic alternating nystagmus	Cervicomedullary junction	Multiple sclerosis, cranial malformation
Seesaw nystagmus	Anterior third ventricle	Neoplasm
Convergence-retractory nystagmus	Dorsal midbrain	Neoplasm, multiple sclerosis
Ocular myoclonus	Dentatorubro-olivary triangle	Infarction, multiple sclerosis
Ocular flutter and opsoclonus	Cerebellar pathways	Brainstem or cerebellar encephalitis, occult neuroblastoma
Ocular bobbing	Pons	Infarction, toxic or metabolic encephalopathy

Endocrine paraneoplastic syndromes

Syndrome	Mediator	Associated malignancy
Hypercalcemia	Parathyroid hormone (parathormone, PTH) or PTH-like substance	Breast cancer
		Squamous cell carcinoma of lung, head and neck, esophagus
	Osteoclast-activating factors	Multiple myeloma
	Prostaglandins	Renal cell carcinoma
	Tumor growth factor (TGF), alpha	
	Interleukin-1 (IL-1)	
	Tumor necrosis factor	
	Lymphotoxin	
Syndrome of inappropriate secretion of antidiuretic hormone (SIADH)	Antidiuretic hormone (ADH)	Small cell carcinoma of lung
		Head and neck carcinomas
		Hodgkin's disease
		Non-Hodgkin's lymphoma
Hypoglycemia	Insulin	Insulinoma
	Insulin-like peptides	Mesenchymal tumors, including mesothelioma, fibrosarcoma, neurofibrosarcoma, rhabdomyosarcoma
Zollinger-Ellison syndrome	Gastrin	Gastrinoma
Ectopic secretion of human chorionic gonadotropin	Human chorionic gonadotropin (HCG)	Germ cell tumors containing trophoblastic elements
Cushing's syndrome	Adrenocorticotropic hormone (ACTH)	Lung carcinoma

Differential diagnosis of parkinsonism

Idiopathic Parkinson's disease

Systems degeneration (Parkinson's-plus syndromes)

Progressive supranuclear palsy
Shy-Drager syndrome
Olivopontocerebellar atrophy
Striatonigral degeneration
Cortical-basal ganglionic degeneration
Huntington's disease (rigid variant)
Wilson's disease
Alzheimer's disease with extrapyramidal rigidity

Secondary parkinsonism

Postencephalitic parkinsonism
  Drug-induced parkinsonism
  Cerebrovascular disease
    Binswanger's disease
    Basal ganglia lacunes
  Normal pressure hydrocephalus
  Trauma, midbrain injury
  Tumor, vascular malformation (rare)
  Toxic/metabolic
    N-methyl-4-phenyl-tetrahydropyridine (MPTP)
    Manganese
    Carbon monoxide poisoning
    Non-Wilsonian hepatocerebral degeneration
    Hyperparathyroidism

Differential diagnosis of clinical features of pulmonary embolism

Dyspnea

Atelectasis
Pneumonia
Pneumothorax
Acute pulmonary edema
Acute bronchitis
Acute bronchiolitis
Acute bronchial obstruction

Acute right-sided heart failure

Myocardial infarction
Myocarditis
Cardiac tamponade
Acute respiratory infection
Complicating chronic lung disease

Pleuritic chest pain

Pneumonia
Pneumothorax
Pericarditis
Pulmonary neoplasm
Bronchiectasis
Subdiaphragmatic inflammation
Myositis
Muscle strain
Rib fracture

Cardiovascular collapse

Myocardial infarction
Acute massive hemorrhage
Gram-negative septicemia
Cardiac tamponade
Spontaneous pneumothorax

Hemoptysis

Pneumonia
Bronchial neoplasm
Bronchiectasis
Acute bronchitis
Mitral stenosis
Tuberculosis

Patterns of pulmonary function abnormalities in various pulmonary diseases

Patterns of abnormalities	VC	RV	TLC	FEV_1/FVC	D_LCO
Obstructive					
Asthma	N or ↓	N or ↑	N or ↑	↓	N or ↑
Chronic bronchitis	N or ↓	N or ↑	N	↓	N
Emphysema	N or ↓	↑	↑	↓	↓
Restrictive					
Pulmonary parenchyma	↓	↓	↓	N or ↑	↓
Extrapulmonary	↓	↓	↓	N	N
Restrictive and obstructive diseases	↓	N or ↓	↓	↓	N or ↓

VC, vital capacity; RV, residual volume; TLC, total lung capacity; FEV_1, forced expiratory volume in 1 second; FVC, forced vital capacity; D_LCO, diffusing capacity of carbon monoxide; N, normal; ↓, decreased; ↑, increased.

Causes of solitary pulmonary nodules

Cause	Range of reported incidence (%)
Malignant tumors	
Bronchogenic carcinoma	16-52
Bronchial adenoma (certain cell types seem benign and have benign courses)	1-2
Metastatic carcinoma	1-10
Benign tumors	5-12
Hamartoma	1-2
Fibroma	0-1
Granulomas	
Histoplasmosis	5-38
Tuberculosis	10-15
Coccidioidomycosis	2-14
Cryptococcosis	0-1
Miscellaneous	
Bronchogenic cyst	1-3
Arteriovenous malformation	0-1
Bronchopulmonary sequestration	0-1
Sclerosing hemangioma	0-1
Intrapulmonary lymph node	0-1

Pulmonary nodule, solitary

SIADH

Differential diagnosis of the syndrome of inappropriate antidiuretic hormone (SIADH) secretion

Neoplasms
   Lung (small cell in 80%), pancreas, duodenum, lymphoma, ureter, prostate, Ewing's sarcoma
Pulmonary
   Infection (viral, bacterial, fungal), abscess, asthma, respirator therapy
Central nervous system
   Trauma, neoplasms, infections, vascular, degenerative diseases (including aging), psychoses
Cardiac
   Atrial tachycardias, post-mitral-commissurotomy syndrome
Metabolic
   Myxedema, adrenal insufficiency, acute porphyria, anterior pituitary insufficiency, angiotensin II
Stress
Drugs
   Hypoglycemic agents (chlorpropamide, tolbutamide), antineoplastic drugs (cyclophosphamide, vincristine), narcotics (morphine, barbiturates), psychotropics (phenothiazine derivatives)

Vulvovaginitis

Clinical and laboratory finding	Trichomoniasis	Candidiasis	Bacterial vaginosis
Symptoms			
Pruritus	+++	+++	+
Discharge	+++	+	++
Odor	+	+	+++
Menses	Increased after	Increased before	Not related
Discharge			
	Thin, purulent	Thick, adherent	Thin, adherent
Froth	++		+
Color	White, yellow, green	White	Grayish white
pH	Elevated	4.5	Elevated
Whiff test	++		++++
Microscopy			
Flora	Rods or coccobacilli	Rods, yeasts, pseudohyphae	Coccobacilli
PMNs	+++	May be present	
Epithelial cells	Normal	Normal	Clue cells

Classification of Disease Processes

Classification of acute abdominal pain

A. Urgent condition
   1. Appendicitis
   2. Abdominal aortic aneurysm
      a. Ruptured aneurysm
      b. Dissecting aneurysm
   3. Perforation
      a. Peptic ulcer (stomach, duodenum)
      b. Diverticulum of colon
      c. Meckel's diverticulum
      d. Diverticulum of duodenum, small intestine
      e. Duodenal stump (after gastric resection)
      f. Surgical anastomosis
      g. Boerhaave syndrome
      h. Crohn's disease
      i. Ingested foreign body (chicken bone, straight pin, etc.)
      j. Cecal volvulus
      k. Nonspecific ulcers of jejunum or ileum
      l. Lymphoma (especially *after* therapy)
      m. Gallbladder
      n. Ulcerative colitis (with toxic dilatation)
   4. Obstruction with strangulated loop of bowel
      a. Adhesions
      b. Hernias
      c. Cecal or sigmoid volvulus
      d. Gastric volvulus
   5. Ischemia of small intestine
      a. Occlusive ischemia
      b. Nonocclusive ischemia
   6. Acute cholecystitis, cholangitis
   7. Ruptured ectopic pregnancy
   8. Bacterial abscess of liver
   9. Pancreatic abscess
   10. Ruptured hepatic adenoma, hepatoma, or hemangioma
   11. Ruptured spleen

Classification of acute abdominal pain—cont'd

B. Less urgent condition
   1. Viral gastroenteritis
   2. Staphylococcal toxin gastroenteritis
   3. Peptic ulcer
   4. Hepatitis
      a. Viral
      b. Toxic
      c. Ischemic
   5. Spontaneous bacterial peritonitis
   6. Acute pancreatitis
   7. Diabetic neuropathy
   8. Crohn's disease
   9. Ulcerative colitis
   10. Pelvic inflammatory disease
   11. Infectious enterocolitis
   12. Mesenteric lymphadenitis
   13. Nephroureterolithiasis
   14. Budd-Chiari syndrome
   15. Veno-occlusive disease of liver
   16. Splenic infarction
   17. Twisted ovarian cyst
   18. Hemorrhage into uterine fibroid
   19. Fitz-Hugh–Curtis syndrome
   20. Endometritis
   21. Psychogenic
   22. Diverticulitis
   23. Intestinal obstruction
   24. Skeletal muscle spasm, hematoma, tear
C. Deceptive causes of abdominal pain
   1. Myocardial infarction
   2. Pulmonary embolus
   3. Adrenal insufficiency
   4. Herpes zoster
   5. Acute pyelonephritis
   6. Pneumonia
   7. Trauma to testicle
   8. Familial Mediterranean fever
   9. Porphyria

Classification of aplastic anemia by cause

Idiopathic
Drugs
    Chloramphenicol
    Phenylbutazone and related anti-inflammatory drugs
    Quinacrine and related antiprotozoals
    Sulfonamides
    Cimetidine
    Gold salts
    Hydantoins
Chemicals
    Benzene and benzene-containing solvents
    Insecticides including DDT
Viral
    Hepatitis
    Epstein-Barr virus
    Human immunodeficiency virus
Immunologic
    Graft-versus-host disease
    Systemic lupus erythematosus
    Eosinophilic fasciitis
    Thymoma
Pregnancy
Congenital
    Fanconi anemia
    Dyskeratosis congenita
    Shwachman-Diamond syndrome
    Reticular dysgenesis

Megaloblastic anemias

I. Etiopathophysiologic classification of cobalamin (Cbl) deficiency
   A. Nutritional Cbl deficiency (insufficient Cbl intake) vegetarians, vegans, breast-fed infants of mothers with pernicious anemia
   B. Abnormal intragastric events (inadequate proteolysis of food Cbl) atrophic gastritis, partial gastrectomy with hypochlorhydria
   C. Loss/atrophy of gastric oxyntic mucosa (deficient IF molecules) total or partial gastrectomy, pernicious anemia (PA), caustic destruction (lye)
   D. Abnormal events in small bowel lumen
      1. Inadequate pancreatic protease (R-Cbl not degraded, Cbl not transferred to IF)
         (i) Insufficiency of pancreatic protease — pancreatic insufficiency
         (ii) Inactivation of pancreatic protease — Zollinger-Ellison syndrome
      2. Usurping of luminal Cbl (inadequate Cbl binding to IF)
         (i) By bacteria — stasis syndromes (blind loops, pouches of diverticulosis, strictures, fistulas, anastomoses); impaired bowel motility (scleroderma, pseudo-obstruction), hypogammaglobulinemia
         (ii) By *Diphyllobothrium latum*
   E. Disorders of ileal mucosa/IF receptors (IF-Cbl not bound to IF receptors)
      1. Diminished or absent IF receptors — ileal bypass/resection/fistula
      2. Abnormal mucosal architecture/function — tropical/nontropical sprue, Crohn's disease, TB ileitis, infiltration by lymphomas, amyloidosis
      3. IF-/post IF-receptor defects — Immerslund-Gräsbeck syndrome, TC II deficiency
      4. Drug-induced effects (slow K, biguanides, cholestyramine, colchicine, neomycin, PAS)
   F. Disorders of plasma Cbl transport (TC II-Cbl not delivered to TC II receptors)
      1. Congenital TC II deficiency, defective binding of TC II-Cbl to TC II receptors (rare)
   G. Metabolic disorders (Cbl not utilized by cell)
      1. Inborn enzyme errors (rare)
      2. Acquired disorders: (Cbl oxidized to cob[III]alamin) — N_2O inhalation   *Continued.*

Megaloblastic anemias—cont'd

II. Etiopathophysiologic classification of folate deficiency
   A. Nutritional causes
      1. Decrease dietary intake—poverty and famine (associated with kwashiorkor, marasmus)/institutionalized individuals (psychiatric/nursing homes)/chronic debilitating disease/ goat's milk (low in folate), special diets (slimming)/ cultural/ethnic cooking techniques (food folate destroyed) or habits (folate-rich foods not consumed)
      2. Decreased diet and increased requirements
         (i) *Physiologic:* pregnancy and lactation, prematurity, infancy
         (ii) *Pathologic:* intrinsic hematologic disease (autoimmune hemolytic disease, drugs, malaria; hemoglobinopathies (SS, thalassemia), RBC membrane defects (hereditary spherocytosis, paroxysmal nocturnal hemoglobinopathy); abnormal hematopoiesis (leukemia/ lymphoma, myelodysplastic syndrome, agnogenic myeloid metaplasia with myelofibrosis); infiltration with malignant disease; dermatologic—psoriasis
   B. Folate malabsorption
      1. With normal intestinal mucosa
         (i) Some drugs (controversial)
         (ii) Congenital folate malabsorption (rare)
      2. With mucosal abnormalities—tropical and nontropical sprue, regional enteritis
   C. Defective cellular folate uptake—familial aplastic anemia (rare)
   D. Inadequate cellular utilization
      1. Folate antagonists (methotrexate)
      2. Hereditary enzyme deficiencies involving folate
   E. Drugs (multiple effects on folate metabolism)—alcohol, sulfasalazine, triamterine, pyrimethamine, trimethoprim-sulfamethoxazole, diphenylhydantoin, barbiturates
   F. Acute folate deficiency
III. Miscellaneous megaloblastic anemias (not caused by Cbl or folate deficiency)
   A. Congenital disorders of DNA synthesis (rare)-orotic aciduria, Lesch-Nyhan syndrome, congenital dyserythropoietic anemia
   B. Acquired disorders of DNA synthesis
      1. Thiamine-responsive megaloblastosis (rare)
      2. Malignancy—erythroleukemia
                           —refractory sideroblastic anemias
                           —*all* antineoplastic drugs that inhibit DNA synthesis
      3. Toxic-alcohol

Classification of disorders causing low back pain

Lumbar disk syndromes
    L4 nerve root compression
    L5 nerve root compression
    S1 nerve root compression
    Large midline disk herniation
Congenital abnormalities
    Facet asymmetry
    Transitional vertebral (Bertolloti's syndrome)
    Spondylolisthesis-spondylolysis
    Scheuermann's disease
    Achondroplasia
Arthritic conditions
    Hypertrophic arthritis
    Osteoarthritis
    Ankylosing spondylitis
    Rheumatoid arthritis
    Osteitis condensans ilii
Infections
    Acute bacterial disk space infection
    Tuberculous spondylitis
    Sacroiliac infection
Tumors
    Benign
        Meningioma or neurinoma
        Osteoid osteoma
        Osteoblastoma
    Malignant
        Metastatic cancer (breast, lung, prostate, etc.)
        Primary neural tumors
        Myelogenous diseases
            Multiple myeloma
            Hodgkin's disease
            Lymphoma
            Eosinophilic granuloma
            Hand-Schüller-Christian syndrome
Metabolic disease
    Osteoporosis
    Ochronosis
    Paget's disease
    Sickle cell disease
Trauma
    Lumbar strain
    Compression fracture
    Subluxation of facet joint   *Continued.*

Classification of disorders causing low back pain—cont'd

Nonskeletal disorders
   Myofascial pain
   Pelvic disorders (pelvic inflammatory disease, uterine fibroids, tumors)
   Ectopic pregnancy
   Retroperitoneal tumors or hematoma
   Prostatitis
   Abdominal aortic aneurysm
   Kidney stones
   Pyelonephritis
   Pancreatitis
   Peptic ulcer
   Large bowel obstruction

Classification of cardiac failure

I. Mechanical abnormalities
   A. Increased resistance to forward outflow (pressure overload)
   B. Increased ventricular inflow (volume overload): valvular regurgitation, shunts, increased blood volume
      1. Primary
      2. Secondary (valvular regurgitation from ventricular dilatation)
   C. Pericardial disease (constriction and tamponade)
   D. Restrictive heart disease (endocardial or myocardial)
   E. Ventricular aneurysm
II. Myocardial failure
   A. Primary
      1. Cardiomyopathy
      2. Myocarditis
      3. Metabolically induced muscle dysfunction (hypothyroidism)
      4. Reduction in muscle mass (myocardial infarction)
   B. Secondary
      1. Dysdynamic heart failure (longstanding volume or pressure overload)
      2. Drug induced
      3. Cardiac involvement in systemic disease
III. Electrical disorders
   A. Asystole
   B. Ventricular fibrillation
   C. Heart block
   D. Ventricular tachycardia

Classification of diuretics by site of action in the nephron

Osmotic diuretics
   Urea
   Mannitol
Proximal tubular diuretics
   Mannitol
   Acetazolamide
Loop of Henle diuretics
   Ethacrynic acid
   Furosemide
   Bumetanide
Distal tubular diuretics
   Potassium-losing diuretics
      Thiazides
      Chlorthalidone
      Metolazone
      Indapamide
   Potassium-sparing diuretics
      Triamterene
      Spironolactone
      Amiloride

Classification of epileptic seizures

Generalized (no detectable focus)
   Tonic-clonic (grand mal)
   Absence (petit mal)
   Tonic
   Myoclonic
   Clonic
   Akinetic
Partial (focal onset)
   Simple (consciousness intact)
      Motor
      Sensory
      Autonomic
      Psychic
   Complex (consciousness impaired)
      Simple onset, with later impairment of consciousness
      Impaired consciousness at onset
   Partial evolving to secondarily generalized convulsion

Classification of gallstones

	Cholesterol	Polymer calcium (hydrogen) bilirubinate ("black") pigment	Calcium (hydrogen) bilirubinate ("brown") pigment
Primary location	Gallbladder	Gallbladder	90% biliary tree 10% gallbladder*
Number	Solitary (~10%) Multiple (90%)	Multiple	Solitary or multiple
Size	Up to 4 cm	2 to 5 mm	2 to 20 mm
Appearance	White–Yellow–Brown	Shiny black	Earthy brown
Hardness	Hard	Hard	Soft
Clinical associations	Hypersecretion of biliary cholesterol	Increased bilirubin secretion and bile salt deficiency	Anaerobic biliary infection and biliary obstruction
Cholesterol content	> 70%	0–10%	< 30%
Calcium salts	Calcium carbonate or phosphate	Calcium phosphate carbonate and calcium (hydrogen) bilirubinate	Calcium (fatty acid) soaps, calcium (hydrogen) bilirubinate
Radiodensity	Lucent or rim calcification	70% opaque	Lucent

*Most likely secondary to prior episodes of healed, acute cholecystitis.

Chronic hepatitis summary

Type	Etiology	Histologic subgroups	Prognosis	Treatment
Chronic persistent hepatitis	Autoimmune hepatitis (AIH) Hepatitis B virus Hepatitis C virus Hepatitis D virus Drugs	Chronic persistent hepatitis Unresolved acute hepatitis	Benign*	Reassurance and periodic follow-up for AIH Interferon alpha-2b for hepatitis B, ? for hepatitis C Withdraw potentially offending drugs

Chronic active hepatitis	Autoimmune hepatitis (AIH)
	Hepatitis B virus
	Hepatitis C virus
	Hepatitis D virus
	Drugs (isoniazid, methyldopa, nitrofurantoin)
		1. Chronic active hepatitis without cirrhosis
		  a. Piecemeal necrosis only
		  b. Bridging hepatic necrosis or multilobular necrosis
		
		2. Chronic active hepatitis with cirrhosis
		
		3. Inactive cirrhosis
			1a. Probably not precirrhotic†
			  b. Definitely precirrhotic
			
			2. Already cirrhotic
			
			3. Already cirrhotic
				1a. Reassurance and periodic follow-up for AIH; interferon alpha-2b for hepatitis B and C
				  b. Prednisone and Azathioprine for AIH; interferon alpha-2b for hepatitis B and C
				
				2. Prednisone and azathioprine for AIH; interferon alpha-2b for hepatitis B and C
				
				3. Careful follow-up;
				  Withdraw potentially offending drugs

*An unknown percentage of patients with chronic persistent hepatitis C will progress to CAH and cirrhosis.
†An unknown percentage of patients with chronic active hepatitis B and C will progress to CAH and cirrhosis.

Types of hypertension

I. Systolic and diastolic hypertension
  A. Primary, essential, or idiopathic
  B. Secondary
    1. Renal
      a. Renal parenchymal disease
        (1) Acute glomerulonephritis
        (2) Chronic nephritis
        (3) Polycystic disease
        (4) Connective tissue diseases
        (5) Diabetic nephropathy
        (6) Hydronephrosis
      b. Renovascular
      c. Renin-producing tumors
      d. Renoprival
      e. Primary sodium retention (Liddle's syndrome, Gordon's syndrome)
    2. Endocrine
      a. Acromegaly
      b. Hypothyroidism
      c. Hyperthyroidism
      d. Hypercalcemia (hyperparathyroidism)
      e. Adrenal
        (1) Cortical
          (a) Cushing's syndrome
          (b) Primary aldosteronism
          (c) Congenital adrenal hyperplasia
        (2) Medullary: pheochromocytoma
      f. Extraadrenal chromaffin tumors
      g. Carcinoid
      h. Exogenous hormones
        (1) Estrogen
        (2) Glucocorticoids
        (3) Mineralocorticoids: licorice
        (4) Sympathomimetics
        (5) Tyramine-containing foods and monoamine oxidase inhibitors

Types of hypertension—cont'd

3. Coarctation of the aorta
4. Pregnancy-induced hypertension
5. Neurological disorders
    a. Increased intracranial pressure
        (1) Brain tumor
        (2) Encephalitis
        (3) Respiratory acidosis
    b. Sleep apnea
    c. Quadriplegia
    d. Acute porphyria
    e. Familial dysautonomia
    f. Lead poisoning
    g. Guillain-Barré syndrome
6. Acute stress, including surgery
    a. Psychogenic hyperventilation
    b. Hypoglycemia
    c. Burns
    d. Pancreatitis
    e. Alcohol withdrawal
    f. Sickle cell crisis
    g. Postresuscitation
    h. Postoperative
7. Increased intravascular volume
8. Alcohol, drugs, etc.

II. Systolic hypertension
    A. Increased cardiac output
        1. Aortic valvular regurgitation
        2. Arteriovenous fistula, patent ductus
        3. Thyrotoxicosis
        4. Paget's disease of bone
        5. Beriberi
        6. Hyperkinetic circulation
    B. Rigidity of aorta

From Kaplan NM: Clinical hypertension, ed 5. Baltimore, 1990, Williams & Wilkins.

Classification of hypogonadotropic hypogonadism

I. Organic causes
   A. Multiple tropic hormone deficiencies
      1. Idiopathic
      2. Secondary to tumor
      3. Miscellaneous causes
         a. Histiocytosis X
         b. Tuberculosis
         c. Sarcoidosis
         d. Collagen vascular diseases
         e. Hypophysitis
   B. Secondary to hyperprolactinemia
   C. Isolated gonadotropin deficiency
      1. Hypogonadotropic eunuchoidism (Kallmann's syndrome)
         a. Complete
         b. Partial (predominant LH deficiency—"fertile eunuch syndrome")
         c. Variant form (isolated FSH deficiency)
      2. Specific genetic syndromes
         a. Prader-Labhart-Willi
         b. Laurence-Moon-Biedl
         c. Möbius
         d. Other rarer disorders
   D. Acute and chronic illness
      1. Malnutrition
      2. Miscellaneous acute illnesses
      3. Emotional disorders
      4. Liver disease (one subgroup)
      5. Renal disease (one component)
      6. Hemochromatosis
      7. Human immunodeficiency virus infection
II. Functional cause
   A. Physiologic delayed puberty

Classification and differential diagnosis of intestinal obstruction

   I. Paralytic ileus
  II. Concentric narrowing
     A. Crohn's disease
     B. Neoplasm (lymphoma, adenocarcinoma, other)
     C. Diverticulitis
     D. Resolved ischemic enteritis
 III. Kinking of a loop
     A. Postoperative adhesions
     B. Incarcerated hernia
 IV. Twisting of a loop
     A. Cecal volvulus
     B. Sigmoid volvulus
     C. Midgut volvulus
  V. Intussusception
     A. Spontaneous
     B. Secondary to polyp or mass
 VI. Foreign body
     A. Ingested
     B. Gallstone
VII. Pseudo-obstruction

Classification of intestinal pseudo-obstruction

 I. "Primary" (idiopathic intestinal pseudo-obstruction)
    A. Hollow visceral myopathy
      1. Familial
      2. Sporadic
    B. Neuropathic
      1. Abnormal myenteric plexus
      2. Normal myenteric plexus
II. Secondary
    A. Scleroderma
    B. Myxedema
    C. Amyloidosis
    D. Muscular dystrophy
    E. Hypokalemia
    F. Chronic renal failure
    G. Diabetes mellitus
    H. Drug toxicity caused by
      1. Anticholinergics
      2. Opiate narcotics
    I. Ogilvie's syndrome

Classification of mediastinal masses

Anterior or anterosuperior

Thymoma
Germ cell tumor
Lymphoma
Substernal goiter
Enlarged fat pad or lipoma
Aneurysm of ascending aorta
Parathyroid adenoma

Middle

Bronchogenic carcinoma
Bronchogenic cyst
Lymphoma
Metastatic tumor
Systemic granuloma (sarcoid, histoplasmosis, tuberculosis)
Pericardial cyst

Posterior

Neurogenic tumor
Bronchogenic cyst
Enteric cyst
Aneurysm of descending aorta
Diaphragmatic hernia
Paravertebral abscess
Meningocele
Achalasia

Etiologic classification of myoclonus (after Marsden, Hallett, and Fahn)

Physiologic

Sleep jerks
Hiccup

Essential

Familial essential myoclonus
Sporadic essential myoclonus
Startle syndromes

Epileptic myoclonus (fragments of epilepsy)

Partial continuous epilepsy
Photomyoclonic response
Primary generalized epileptic myoclonus
Juvenile atonic-myoclonic epilepsy (Lennox-Gastaut)
Infantile spasms
Benign myoclonus of infancy
Baltic myoclonus (Unverricht-Lundborg)

Symptomatic myoclonus

Storage disease with progressive myoclonus epilepsy
    Lafora body disease
    Neuronal ceroid lipofuscinosis
    Sialidosis
    Gaucher's disease
    GM_2 gangliosidosis
    Mitochondrial encephalomyopathy (MERRF)
Toxic/metabolic encephalopathy
Spinocerebellar, basal ganglia degenerations
    Friedreich's ataxia
    Wilson's disease
    Progressive supranuclear palsy
    Huntington's disease
Alzheimer's disease
Creutzfeldt-Jacob disease
Viral encephalitis
Posthypoxic (Lance-Adams)
Focal CNS damage
    Palatal myoclonus
    Spinal myoclonus

After Marsden CD, Hallett M, and Fahn S: In Marsden CD and Fahn S, editors: *Movement disorders*. London, 1982, Butterworth Scientific.

Classification of primary myopathies

I. Hereditary
    A. Muscular dystrophies
    B. Congenital myopathies
    C. Metabolic myopathies
       1. Glycogenolysis and glycolysis
          a. Myophosphorylase, phosphofructokinase deficiency
          b. Distal glycolytic enzyme deficiencies
       2. Lipid
          a. Carnitine-palmityl-transferase A or B deficiency
          b. Systemic and muscle carnitine deficiency
          c. Defective beta decarboxylation
       3. Purine
       4. Mitochondria
          a. Defined biochemical defects
          b. Mitochondrial DNA mutations
          c. Mitochondrial DNA depletion (e.g., AZT therapy)
    D. Membrane excitability disorders
       1. Myotonia
          a. Myotonic dystrophy
          b. Myotonia congenita
       2. Periodic paralysis
          a. Sodium channel mutations
             (i) Hyperkalemic periodic paralysis
             (ii) Normokalemic periodic paralysis
             (iii) Paramyotonia congenita
          b. Hypokalemic periodic paralysis
II. Inflammatory
    A. Polymyositis ($\pm$ dermatomyositis)
    B. Polymyositis with vasculitis
    C. Inclusion body myositis
    D. Infectious
       1. Bacterial (e.g., clostridial)
       2. Viral and retroviral (e.g., Coxsackie, HIV)
       3. Parasitic (e.g., toxoplasmosis)
    E. Drug-induced
    F. Miscellaneous (e.g., sarcoidosis, paraneoplastic)
III. Endocrine metabolic
    A. Electrolyte disturbances (e.g., calcium, magnesium, potassium)
    B. Endocrine disturbance
       1. Cushing's disease
       2. Hypo- and hyperthyroidism
       3. Hypo- and hyperparathyroidism
IV. Toxic (e.g., alcohol, steroids, halothane, vincristine, chloroquine)
V. Primary muscle tumors
VI. Miscellaneous (e.g., malignant hyperthermia)

Classification of obesity

Familial
   Onset usually in childhood
   Prevalence in first-degree relatives
   Genetic and cultural determinants
   Potential association with other diseases such as non–insulin dependent diabetes mellitus, hyperlipidemias, hypertension, gout
Isolated
   Onset usually in adolescence or adulthood
   Common contributing factors
      Increased food intake
      Decreased physical activity
      Withdrawal from smoking
      Estrogens
      Drugs affecting energy intake or expenditure
         Phenothiazines, serotonin antagonists tricyclic antidepressants, marijuana, sulfonylureas
   Commonly associated diseases
Hypothalamic disorders
   Tumors—craniopharyngioma, glioma, cyst, etc.
   Inflammation—sarcoidosis, tuberculosis, eosinophilic granuloma, encephalitis, leukemia
   Trauma—after head injury
   Benign intracranial hypertension
Endocrine disorders
   Cushing's syndrome
   Insulinoma
   Hypothyroidism
   Hypogonadism
   Polycystic ovary syndrome
   Growth hormone deficiency
Congenital disorders
   Prader-Willi syndrome
   Laurence-Moon-Biedl syndrome
   Alstrom's syndrome
   Familial partial lipodystrophy

Classification of occlusive arterial disease

I. Acute arterial occlusion
   A. Thrombotic arterial occlusion secondary to
      1. Atherosclerosis
         a. Arteriosclerosis obliterans
         b. Atherosclerotic aneurysm
      2. Thromboangiitis obliterans (Buerger's disease)
      3. Arteritis resulting from
         a. Connective tissue diseases
         b. Giant-cell (temporal or cranial) arteritis
         c. Takayasu's arteritis
      4. Myeloproliferative disease
         a. Polycythemia vera
         b. Thrombocytosis
      5. Hypercoagulable states
         a. Complicating neoplastic disease
         b. Complicating ulcerative bowel disease
         c. Idiopathic ("simple") arterial thrombosis
      6. Trauma
         a. Arterial puncture and arteriotomy
         b. Secondary to fractures and bone dislocations
         c. Arterial entrapment
            (1) Lower extremity
               (a) Adductor tendon compression of superficial
                   femoral artery
               (b) Popliteal artery entrapment
            (2) Upper extremity
               (a) Thoracic outlet compression
               (b) "Crutch" thrombosis
         d. Frostbite
   B. Embolic arterial occlusion (arising from thrombi of)
      1. Cardiac origin
         a. Valvular heart disease, including valvular prostheses
         b. Acute myocardial infarction
         c. Myocardial aneurysm
         d. Atrial fibrillation
         e. Cardiomyopathy
         f. Infective endocarditis
         g. Left-sided myxoma

Classification of occlusive arterial disease—cont'd

   2. Proximal atherosclerotic plaques or arterial narrowing
   3. Proximal arterial aneurysms
      a. Atherosclerotic
      b. Poststenotic dilatation
      c. Fibromuscular dysplasia
   C. Miscellaneous causes
      1. Arterial spasm, secondary to
         a. Ergotism
         b. Trauma of blunt or penetrating type
         c. Intra-arterial injections
      2. Aortic dissection
         a. Luminal compression (by extension of the dissection into branch[es] of the aorta)
         b. Occlusion at site of reentry of dissection
      3. Foreign bodies
         a. Bullet embolism
         b. Guidewires and catheters
II. Chronic arterial occlusive disease
   A. Arteriosclerosis obliterans
   B. Thromboangiitis obliterans (Buerger's disease)
   C. Arteritis
      1. Connective tissue disorders
      2. Giant-cell (temporal or cranial) arteritis
      3. Takayasu's disease
   D. Trauma
      1. Blunt trauma
         a. Chronic occupational arterial occlusion in the hand
      2. Arterial entrapment
         a. Superficial femoral artery
         b. Popliteal artery
   E. Congenital arterial narrowing

From Spittell JA Jr: Office and bedside diagnosis of occlusive arterial disease. Curr Probl Cardiol 8:1, 1983. With permission of Year Book Medical Publishers, Inc.

Classification of osteoarthritis

I. Primary
   A. Idiopathic
   B. Generalized osteoarthritis
   C. Erosive osteoarthritis
II. Secondary
   A. Resulting from mechanical incongruity of joint
      1. Congenital or developmental defects, hip dysplasia, Legg-Calvé-Perthes disease, slipped femoral capital epiphysis, femoral neck abnormalities, protrusio acetabuli, multiple epiphyseal dysplasia, osteochondritis, Morquio's syndrome
      2. Posttraumatic
   B. Resulting from prior inflammatory joint disease—for example, rheumatoid arthritis and variants, chronic gouty arthritis, pseudogout, infectious arthritis
   C. Resulting from metabolic disorders—for example, hemochromatosis, ochronosis, Wilson's disease, chondrocalcinosis, Paget's disease
   D. Resulting from endocrinopathies—for example, diabetes mellitus, acromegaly, sex hormone abnormalities, iatrogenic hyperadrenocorticism
   E. Resulting from miscellaneous causes—for example, osteonecrosis, hemarthrosis associated with blood dyscrasias

Classification of pleural effusions

I. Transudates
    A. Increased hydrostatic pressure
        1. Congestive heart failure
        2. Constrictive pericarditis
        3. Superior vena caval obstruction
    B. Decreased oncotic pressure
        1. Hypoalbuminemia
            a. Nephrotic syndrome
            b. Cirrhosis
        2. Intra-abdominal disease
            a. Cirrhosis with ascites
            b. Peritoneal dialysis
II. Exudates
    A. Infections
        1. Parapneumonic empyema or effusion
        2. Tuberculosis
        3. Fungi
        4. Parasites
        5. Viral
        6. *Mycoplasma*
    B. Neoplasms
        1. Bronchogenic carcinoma
        2. Metastatic carcinoma
        3. Lymphoma and leukemia
        4. Mesothelioma
    C. Pulmonary emboli and infarction
    D. Intra-abdominal disease
        1. Subdiaphragmatic abscess
        2. Pancreatitis
        3. Meigs' syndrome
    E. Connective tissue and hypersensitivity disease
        1. Rheumatoid arthritis
        2. Lupus erythematosus
        3. Dressler's syndrome
        4. Drug reaction
    F. Miscellaneous
        1. Esophageal rupture
        2. Familial Mediterranean fever
        3. Lymphedema
        4. Myxedema
        5. Atelectasis
        6. Uremia
        7. Benign asbestos related
    G. Idiopathic
III. Hemothorax
IV. Lipidic
    A. Chylous
    B. Cholesterol or pseudochylous

A pathophysiologic classification of pulmonary edemas by etiology

I. Alterations in Starling forces
   A. Increased hydrostatic pressure (heart failure, mitral stenosis, ?neurogenic pulmonary edema)
   B. Decreased plasma oncotic pressure (malnutrition, hepatic failure, massive crystalloid infusion)
II. Altered pulmonary microvascular membrane permeability
   A. Shock (septic, ?hemorrhagic, ?neurogenic, ?cardiogenic)
   B. Infections (viral, fungal, tuberculosis, rickettsial)
   C. Multiple trauma (fat embolism, head trauma)
   D. Inhalation injury
      1. Gastric aspiration
      2. Near-drowning
      3. Hydrocarbons
      4. Irritant and poisonous gases (nitrogen dioxide, ammonia, phosgene, chlorine, cadmium, ozone), smoke
      5. Oxygen toxicity
      6. Hypersensitivity pneumonitis
   E. Drug-related (heroin, aspirin, paraquat)
   F. Hematologic disorders (disseminated intravascular coagulation, transfusion, cardiopulmonary bypass, pulmonary embolism)
   G. Metabolic disorder (pancreatitis, ketoacidosis)
   H. Immunologic (systemic lupus erythematosus, Wegener's granulomatosis, Goodpasture's syndrome)
III. Miscellaneous and poorly understood conditions
   A. Uremia
   B. Eclampsia
   C. Radiation pneumonitis
   D. High-altitude pulmonary edema
   E. Reexpansion of unilateral collapsed lung
   F. Idiopathic

Classification of causes of chronic renal failure

 I. Hereditary
   A. Polycystic kidney disease
   B. Familial glomerulonephritis (Alport's syndrome)
   C. Medullary cystic disease
 II. Systemic disease with potential for renal involvement
   A. Diabetes mellitus
   B. Connective tissue disorders
     1. Systemic lupus erythematosus
     2. Polyarteritis nodosa
     3. Scleroderma
     4. Wegener's granulomatosis
   C. Amyloidosis, myeloma kidney, gout
   D. Essential hypertension
III. Primary glomerulonephritis (major progressive types)
   A. Membranous
   B. Membranoproliferative
   C. Focal glomerulosclerosis
 IV. Primary tubulointerstitial renal disease
   A. Reflux nephropathy
   B. Analgesic abuse nephropathy
   C. Renal stone disease and nephrocalcinosis
  V. Primary vascular renal disease
   A. Hypertensive nephrosclerosis
   B. Bilateral renal artery disease
 VI. Obstructive uropathy
   A. Congenital
   B. Stone disease
   C. Prostatic disease

Classification of acute respiratory failure

Category	Example	Mechanism of hypoxemia	Chest x-ray
↓ PaO_2 with normal or ↓ $PaCO_2$			
Preexisting lung disease	Restrictive lung disease (pulmonary fibrosis)	$\dot{V}/\dot{Q}$ mismatch ± shunt	Diffuse interstitial infiltrate
	Asthma (until very severe)	$\dot{V}/\dot{Q}$ mismatch	Clear
No preexisting lung disease required (but could be superimposed on chronic disease)	Adult respiratory distress syndrome	Shunt	Diffuse alveolar-filling infiltrate
	Cardiogenic pulmonary edema	Shunt	Diffuse alveolar-filling infiltrate
	Pulmonary emboli	$\dot{V}/\dot{Q}$ mismatch and shunt	Clear (or localized infiltrate)
	Pneumonia	Shunt	Localized or diffuse alveolar-filling infiltrate
↓ PaO_2 with ↑ $PaCO_2$			
Previous lung disease	COPD	Hypoventilation and $\dot{V}/\dot{Q}$ mismatch	Clear
	Asthma (very severe)	Hypoventilation and $\dot{V}/\dot{Q}$ mismatch	Clear
Normal lungs	Sedative drug overdose	Hypoventilation	Clear
	Neuromuscular disease (e.g., myasthenia gravis, Guillain-Barré syndrome)	Hypoventilation	Clear

Types of syncope

I. Neurogenic syncope
   A. Vasovagal (vasodepression)
   B. Orthostatic hypotension
      1. Occasional normal individuals
      2. Peripheral neuropathy
      3. Medications
      4. Primary autonomic insufficiency
      5. Intravascular volume depletion
   C. Reflex
      1. Cough
      2. Micturation
      3. Acute pain states
      4. Carotid sinus hypersensitivity
II. Cardiogenic syncope
   A. Mechanical
      1. Outflow tract obstruction
      2. Pulmonary hypertension
      3. Congenital heart disease
      4. Myocardial disease
   B. Electrical
      1. Bradyarrhythmias
      2. Tachyarrhythmias

Classification of vasculitic syndromes

Clinical syndrome	Predominant vessels affected
Takayasu arteritis	Large arteries (aorta and primary branches)
Giant-cell (temporal) arteritis	Large and medium-sized arteries (aorta, primary and secondary branches)
Thromboangiitis obliterans (Buerger's disease)	Medium-sized and small muscular arteries (diverse distributions and locations)
Kawasaki disease	
Polyarteritis nodosa	
Allergic angiitis and granulomatosis (Churg-Strauss syndrome)	
Vasculitis in rheumatic disease (e.g., rheumatoid arthritis, Behçet's syndrome)	
Granulomatous angiitis of CNS	
Wegener granulomatosis	
Vasculitis associated with malignancy (e.g., hairy-cell leukemia)	
Hypersensitivity vasculitis (e.g., serum sickness, drug reactions)	Small vessels (arterioles, capillaries, venules)
Henoch-Schönlein purpura	
Mixed cryoglobulinemia	
Hypocomplementemic urticarial vasculitis	
Cutaneous vasculitis associated with other diseases (e.g., biliary cirrhosis, ulcerative colitis)	

Vasospastic disorders

Raynaud's phenomenon
    Primary (Raynaud's disease)
    Secondary
Livedo reticularis
    Primary
    Secondary
Acrocyanosis
Reflex sympathetic dystrophy
Chronic pernio

From Spittell JA Jr and Spittell PC: Diseases of the aorta and peripheral arteries. In Parmley W and Chatterjee K, editors: Cardiology. Philadelphia, 1987, Lippincott. With permission.

Diagnostic Approach

Alcoholism
Anemia
Angina syndromes, noninvasive studies
Angina, unstable
Antinuclear antibodies
Ascites
Bleeding diathesis
Bleeding disorder, acquired platelet or small vessel
    abnormality
Constipation, chronic
CVA, localization patterns
Diabetes insipidus
Diarrhea, acute
Diarrhea, chronic
Dysphagia
Fever, hospital-acquired
Fever, neutropenic patient
Fever, unknown origin (FUO)
Gastrointestinal bleeding, lower
Hematuria
Hypernatremia
Hypokalemia
Hyponatremia
Hypophosphatemia
Jaundice and hepatobiliary disease
Lymphadenopathy, generalized
Lymphadenopathy, localized
Nephrolithiasis
Neutropenia
Neutrophilia
Pleural effusions
Polycythemia
Raynaud's phenomenon
Splenomegaly
Syncope
Thyroid nodule
Tremor
Urinary tract infection

Alcoholism

Diagnostic tests for alcoholism

1. CAGE

		Sensitivity	Specificity
C	Have you tried to *cut down* on your drinking?	75	96*
A	Are you *annoyed* by people telling you to stop drinking?		
G	Do you feel *guilty* about your drinking?		
E	Do you drink on first getting up in the morning *(eye opener)* ?		

2. Laboratory studies

	Sensitivity	Specificity
Elevated GGT	54	76
Increased mean corpuscular volume	63	74
Elevated liver function test (OT, PT) results	37	81

*For two or more yes answers in CAGE. GGT, gamma glutamyl transpeptidase; OT, oxaloacetic transaminase; PT, pyruvic transaminase.

Evaluation of a patient with a decreased hematocrit.

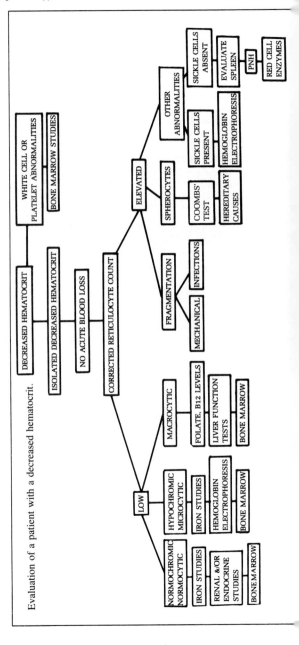

Noninvasive studies in anginal syndromes

1. Classic angina
   a. History, physical examination, and resting ECG
   b. Normal resting ECG: stress electrocardiography to detect high-risk patients or to assess response to therapy
   c. Abnormal resting ECG (uninterpretable): stress thallium myocardial perfusion scan to detect high-risk patients
   d. In patients with poor exercise tolerance: dipyridamole-thallium myocardial perfusion scan to detect severity of coronary artery disease
   e. In patients in whom concurrent assessment of left ventricular function is indicated: resting and exercise gated blood pool scintigraphy or two-dimensional (2D) echocardiography
   f. In patients with previous myocardial infarction and stable angina: stress thallium myocardial perfusion scan (in patients with adequate exercise tolerance) or dipyridamole-thallium myocardial perfusion scan or exercise ventriculography to assess the severity of coronary artery disease and to localize the new vascular territory involved with atherosclerosis
2. Atypical chest pain syndrome
   a. Normal resting ECG: stress electrocardiography
   b. Abnormal resting ECG: stress thallium myocardial perfusion scintigraphy or stress ventriculography (in the absence of other detectable heart disease)
   c. Mitral valve prolapse, chest pain, and abnormal resting ECG: echocardiography and stress thallium myocardial perfusion scintigraphy
   d. Suspected valvular heart disease: 2D echocardiography
3. Variant and unstable angina
   a. History
   b. ECG during chest pain
   c. In patients with prolonged chest pain and uninterpretable ECG: 2D echocardiography; thallium myocardial perfusion scintigraphy and/or gated blood pool scintigraphy

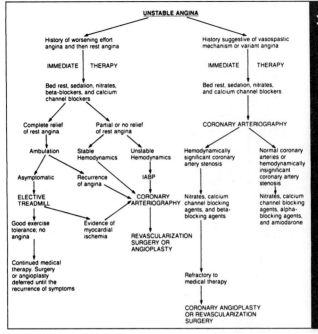

Guidelines for the management of unstable angina. In all patients with unstable angina, aspirin therapy should be considered until it is contraindicated *(not indicated in figure)*. For patients who continue to have rest angina despite antianginal and aspirin therapy, heparin therapy should be considered *(not indicated in figure)*. A few of these patients may also benefit from thrombolytic therapy. *IABP,* Intra-aortic balloon pump.

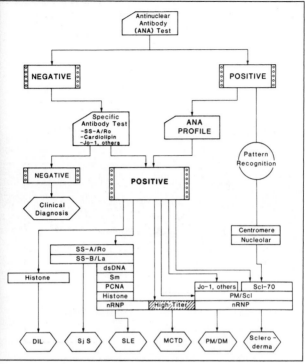

An algorithm showing the diagnostic approach to the use of ANA in the clinical setting. ANA = antinuclear antibodies; DIL = drug-induced lupus; dsDNA = double-stranded DNA; MCTD = mixed connective tissue disease; nRNP = nuclear ribonucleoprotein; PCNA = proliferating cell nuclear antigen (cyclin); PM/DM = polymyositis/dermatomyositis; SjS = Sjögren's syndrome; SLE = systemic lupus erythematosus; SS-A, SS-B = Sjögren's syndrome antigens A,B. (Reprinted from the *Bulletin on the Rheumatic Diseases,* copyright © 1985. Used by permission of the Arthritis Foundation.)

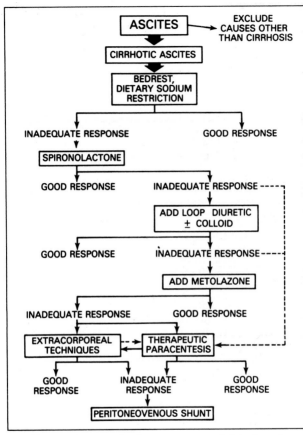

Algorithm for the comprehensive management of cirrhotic ascites and edema. The solid lines represent therapeutic options and sequences that believe are well established. The interrupted lines indicate uncertainty re garding the appropriate positioning of paracentesis in the therapeutic se quence. (Reproduced with permission from Epstein M: Diuretic therapy in liver disease. In Epstein M, editor: The kidney in liver disease, ed 3 Baltimore, 1988, Williams & Wilkins.)

Clinical evaluation of a bleeding patient

I. History
   A. Type of bleeding
      1. Mucocutaneous, petechiae: suggests platelet disorder or vasculitis
      2. Delayed, recurrent oozing; hematoma: suggests plasma coagulation disorder
      3. Menorrhagia or gastrointestinal bleeding possible in either type of disorder
   B. Duration of bleeding
      1. Lifelong: indicates congenital defect of a single factor; confirm with family history of bleeding or presence of consanguinity for suspected recessive traits
      2. Recent onset: indicates an acquired disorder, usually defects of multiple factors; confirm by history of no bleeding with past trauma, surgery, teeth extractions, menses
   C. Systemic illnesses associated with bleeding: liver disease, malignant disease
II. Physical examination
   A. Petechiae and superficial mucocutaneous bleeding
      1. Dependent distribution, asymptomatic: indicates thrombocytopenia
      2. Clusters of palpable, pruritic petechiae: indicates vasculitis
   B. Deep hematomas or hemarthroses, which may be associated with extensive superficial purpura: indicates a coagulation disorder

Clinical evaluation of a bleeding patient—cont'd

III. Preliminary diagnostic categories
    A. Mucocutaneous bleeding, platelet-vessel defect
        1. Congenital
            a. von Willebrand's disease most likely
            b. Well-defined platelet function defects rare; mild, poorly defined platelet defects possibly more common
            c. Thrombocytopenia rare
            d. Afibrinogenemia rare
        2. Acquired
            a. Severe thrombocytopenia most likely caused by auto-immune thrombocytopenic purpura (ITP)
            b. Mild or moderate thrombocytopenia caused by splenic pooling in liver disease common
            c. Other thrombocytopenias caused by peripheral destruction (thrombotic thrombocytopenic purpura, disseminated intravascular coagulation [DIC], sepsis) or marrow failure less common
            d. Mild congenital von Willebrand's disease possible in an adult.
    B. Hematomas and delayed bleeding, coagulation defect
        1. Congenital
            a. Hemophilia A most likely, hemophilia B one-tenth as frequent
            b. Other coagulation defects rare
            c. Homozygous von Willebrand's disease with severe factor VIII deficiency rare
        2. Acquired
            a. Liver disease common
            b. DIC, vitamin K deficiency, coagulation factor inhibitors, anticoagulant therapy
            c. Mild congenital hemophilia possible in an adult
IV. Proceed to laboratory evaluation

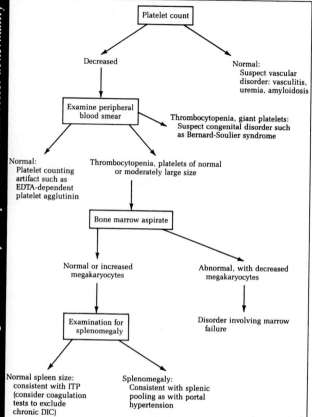

A diagram for the laboratory evaluation of a patient with a bleeding disorder in whom the history and physical examination suggest an acquired disorder of platelets or small vessels.

Approach to the patient with chronic constipation

1. Systemic disease?
   a. Often suggested by physical examination or by history
   b. Helpful laboratory tests include: electrolytes, BUN, tests of thyroid function, calcium, blood sugar
2. History of
   a. Bed rest
   b. Spinal cord lesion
   c. Autonomic neuropathy
   d. Peripheral neuropathy
3. Drug history: stop all potentially constipating drugs
4. Assessment of gastrointestinal tract
   a. Rectal examination
      (1) Tight sphincter, empty ampulla (Hirschsprung's disease)
      (2) Anal and perianal disease (thrombosed hemorrhoid, fissure, fistulas, or abscess)
         (a) Treat and observe
         (b) Rule out associated Crohn's disease if perianal disease is present
      (3) Blood in stool: proceed to flexible sigmoidoscopy and barium studies or colonoscopy
   b. Flexible sigmoidoscopy
      (1) Normal mucosa: proceed to barium enema
      (2) Abnormal: carcinoma, polyp, etc: proceed with colonoscopy
   c. Barium studies or colonoscopy to rule out
      (1) Obstructing lesion (carcinoma, polyp, diverticular mass)
      (2) Stricture (neoplasm, inflammatory bowel disease, ischemia, radiation)
      (3) Short-segment Hirschsprung's disease
      (4) Small intestinal series if barium enema or colonoscopy normal to evaluate for small intestinal obstruction
   d. If cause of either an obstructing mass or stricture is not clear, perform colonoscopy for visual identification and biopsy
   e. If evidence for Hirschsprung's disease or if continued severe idiopathic constipation poorly responsive to medical therapy, perform anal manometry
   f. If no evidence of anal manometry abnormalities and no response to medical management, consider physiologic studies of colonic motility

Common localization patterns

Brain locale or syndrome	Vessels	Findings
1. Left hemisphere anterior circulation	Left ICA, MCA, ACA	Aphasia, right-limb and -face weakness and/or sensory loss, right visual inattention
2. Right hemisphere anterior circulation	Right ICA, MCA, ACA	Left visual neglect, left-limb and -face weakness and/or numbness, poor drawing and copying, lack of recognition of deficit
3. Left occipitotemporal	Left PCA	Right hemianopsia, inability to read but not write and spell, no limb weakness, occasional right hemisensory loss
4. Right occipitotemporal	Right PCA	Left hemianopsia, occasional left hemisensory loss, occasional left neglect
5. Brainstem-cerebellum	Vertebral and basilar arteries	Vertigo, bilateral visual loss, quadraparesis, ataxia, crossed signs (cranial nerves on one side, limb weakness or sensory loss on other side), nystagmus
6. Pure motor stroke (internal capsule in pons)	Penetrating artery	Hemiparesis without cognitive, sensory, or visual loss
7. Pure sensory stroke (thalamus or postlimb internal capsule)	Penetrating artery	Hemisensory symptoms without motor, cognitive, or visual abnormalities

ICA, internal carotid artery; MCA, middle cerebral artery; ACA, anterior cerebral artery; PCA, posterior cerebral artery.

Evaluation of suspected diabetes insipidus

1. Measure plasma osmolality and/or sodium concentration under conditions of ad libitum fluid intake. If they are above 295 mOsm/kg and 143 mEq/L, the diagnosis of primary polydipsia is excluded, and the testing should proceed directly to step 3 to distinguish between neurogenic and nephrogenic diabetes insipidus

2. If basal plasma osmolality and/or sodium is not elevated, perform a dehydration test. If urinary concentration does not occur before plasma osmolality and/or sodium reaches 295 mOsm/kg or 143 mEq/L, the diagnosis of primary polydipsia is again excluded, and the evaluation should proceed to step 3

3. Inject aqueous vasopressin (Pitressin) in a dose of 10 mU/kg body weight and collect urine every 30 minutes for the next 2 hours. If urine osmolality rises more than 50% above the value obtained at the end of the dehydration test, neurogenic diabetes insipidus is established. If not, administer a larger dose of vasopressin (50 mU/kg) to distinguish partial from complete nephrogenic diabetes insipidus

4. If dehydration results in urinary concentration, measure plasma vasopressin level and relate it to concurrent plasma level and to urine osmolality level by using suitable nomograms. If the level of plasma osmolality achieved is insufficient to permit a clear distinction between normal and subnormal vasopressin response (>292 mOsm/kg), infuse 3% saline solution at a rate of 0.1 ml/kg/min for 2 hours, and repeat the measurements of plasma osmolality and vasopressin level

5. If vasopressin level measurements are not available, admit the patient and perform a closely monitored therapeutic trial with intranasal desmopressin, 25 μ every 12 hours. If the trial corrects polydipsia as well as polyuria, and hyponatremia does not occur, the diagnosis of neurogenic diabetes insipidus is established. If the trial reduces polyuria, but not polydipsia, or produces other evidence of water intoxication, primary polydipsia is likely, and therapy should be discontinued until definitive diagnosis can be made by vasopressin assay. If desopressin does not reduce either polyuria or polydipsia, the diagnosis of nephrogenic diabetes insipidus is established. In some patients, repeat tests with higher doses of the drug may be indicated to distinguish between the complete and incomplete forms of the disorder

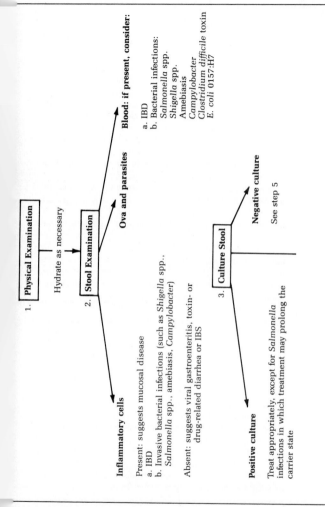

Diagnostic steps in the assessment of acute diarrhea. IBD, inflammatory bowel disease; IBS, irritable bowel syndrome.

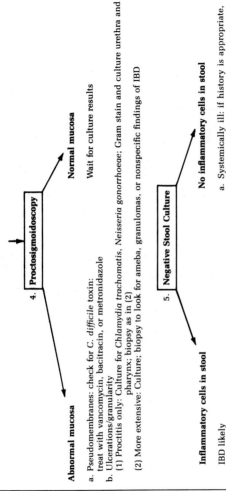

4. **Proctosigmoidoscopy**

Abnormal mucosa

a. Pseudomembranes: check for *C. difficile* toxin: treat with vancomycin, bacitracin, or metronidazole
b. Ulcerations/granularity

   (1) Proctitis only: Culture for *Chlamydia trachomatis, Neisseria gonorrhoeae;* Gram stain and culture urethra and pharynx; biopsy as in (2)

   (2) More extensive: Culture; biopsy to look for ameba, granulomas, or nonspecific findings of IBD

Normal mucosa

Wait for culture results

5. **Negative Stool Culture**

Inflammatory cells in stool

IBD likely

a. Severely ill: rule out toxic megacolon; analyze blood cultures; abdominal x-ray; treat as IBD
b. Not severely ill: barium studies or colonoscopy after careful and gentle preparation

No inflammatory cells in stool

a. Systemically ill: if history is appropriate, with travel to endemic areas, or if patient has hypogammaglobulinemia, evaluate duodenal aspirate for *Giardia*
b. Not systemically ill: stop all drugs, stop milk products, rule out malabsorption, observe, and treat symptomatically; if symptoms persist or recur, perform barium studies or colonoscopy

1. **Diagnostic Steps 1 to 4 as in Fig. 39-1**

   a. Results diagnostic for infectious diarrhea, inflammatory bowel
      disease, or overt drug-induced diarrhea
   b. Results nondiagnostic; usually without inflammatory cells
      in stool

2. **Stool Volume**

   a. Small volume: usually seen in infectious diarrhea or
      inflammatory bowel disease, but can also be seen in
      malabsorption syndromes and irritable bowel syndrome
   b. Large volume: suggests malabsorption syndromes, secretory
      diarrhea, or laxative abuse

3. **Stool Sudan Stain**

Positive ◄—   —► **Negative**

Suggests malabsorption syndrome; pancreatic   See step 4
insufficiency; bile salt insufficiency; or
mucosal disease

Further studies, see Chaps. 31 and 40

4. **Oral Intake Stopped**

Diarrhea continues ◄—   —► **Diarrhea stops**

a. Secretory diarrhea: stool osmolality = stool
   $(Na^+ + K^+) \times 2$
b. Nasogastric suction
   (1) Diarrhea stops
      (a) Zollinger-Ellison syndrome: gastric
          analysis, gastrin, secretin stimulation
      (b) Laxative abuse: see step 5
   (2) Diarrhea continues
      (a) Secretory diarrhea: plasma VIP,
          calcitonin, urinary 5-HIAA
          abdominal ultrasound, computed
          tomography and/or selective mesenteric
          angiogram to identify tumor
      (b) Laxative abuse: see step 5

a. Malabsorption syndromes:
   stool osmolality
   > plasma osmolality
b. Laxative ingestion:
   see step 5
c. Congenital chloridorrhea
   (1) Stool electrolytes:
      chloride concentration
      greater than the sum
      of sodium and potas-
      sium concentration
      in stool water
   (2) No fecal osmotic gap

Diagnostic approach to the patient with chronic diarrhea. VIP, vasoactive
intestinal polypeptide; 5-HIAA, 5-hydroxyindoleacetic acid.

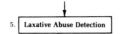

5. **Laxative Abuse Detection**

a. Screening tests
  (1) Locker search
  (2) Add alkali to stool or urine (turns red or pink if phenolphthalein present)
  (3) Sigmoidoscopy for melanosis coli
  (4) Barium enema: dilated, hypomotile "cathartic colon"
b. Specific tests
  (1) Urine screening test for senna
  (2) Chromatographic test for bisacodyl
  (3) Stool test for fecal sulfate and phosphate
  (4) Magnesium concentration in fecal water (atomic absorption spectrophotometry)

6. **Radiologic Studies**

Perform barium studies only after stool examination, culture, and studies requiring quantitative measurements of the stool have been completed.

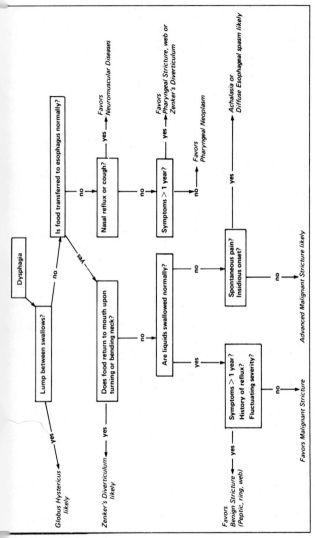

An algorithm for the historical evaluation of dysphagia. (Adapted from D. A. W. Edwards, Flow charts, diagnostic keys and algorithms in the diagnosis of dysphagia. *Scott Med. J.* 15:378, 1970.)

Work flow approach to history and physical examination in diagnosis of hospital-acquired fever

History

—What procedures, instrumentations, or other interventions have been performed since this patient was hospitalized? Has anesthesia been administered?

—What new medications, immunoglobulins, or transfusion products has the patient received since hospitalization?

—Has the patient been treated with antipyretics or other drugs that affect fever?

—Have contrast dyes or other diagnostic products been administered as part of imaging or other diagnostic procedures?

—What underlying diseases has the patient that may be manifested by intermittent fever, which may have created the false appearance of fever as nosocomial?

—Has the patient manifested new symptoms that may signal acquisition of a likely nosocomial pathogen (e.g., nosocomial diarrhea as a manifestation of *Clostridium difficile* infection, sputum production as a manifestation of nosocomial pneumonia)?

Physical examination

Head

—Nasogastric or gastric tube in place? Evaluate for sinusitis.

Chest

—On ventilator now or recently? Operative procedure with general anesthesia since admission?

—New onset or change in character of sputum production or of respiratory function? Careful chest examination for infection or inflammation, follow-up diagnostic studies (radiograph, scanning, etc.) as warranted.

—Murmur or other sign of cardiac dysfunction? If operative or invasive diagnostic procedure performed, evaluate possibility of endocarditis, especially if prophylaxis for the procedure was suboptimum. Blood culture evaluation should be made if there is any suspicion that the fever represents bloodstream invasion.

—Are the patient's prior course and care consistent with a focus for pulmonary emboli?   *Continued.*

Work flow approach to history and physical examination in diagnosis of hospital-acquired fever—cont'd

Physical examination—cont'd

Gastrointestinal

—Onset of diarrhea in the hospital? Evaluate for *Clostridium difficile* infection, especially if the patient has recently been treated with antimicrobial agents. Perhaps more likely, which new medication could be causing local irritation of the gut?

Genital

—Urinary catheter in place now or recently? Obtain urine specimen for microscopic examination (pyuria, hematuria, bacteriuria); if appropriate, follow with Gram's stain and culture.

Operative site or site of trauma

—Signs of superficial or deep infection? Possibility of loculated areas requiring imaging techniques for evaluation?

Extremities

—Are signs of thrombophlebitis or manifestations of extremity ischemia present?

Skin

—Skin rashes are probably the most common and easily noted manifestations of febrile drug reaction, transfusion reaction, and viral or other infections

—Intravascular therapy administered now or recently? Examine closely for phlebitis or exudate at the site of cannulation. Attempt to milk fluid back from vein, and palpate for possible septic thrombophlebitis. Examine fluid container for cracks or cloudy fluid.

—Signs of decubitus or other ulcer, especially one that has broken down since hospital stay began?

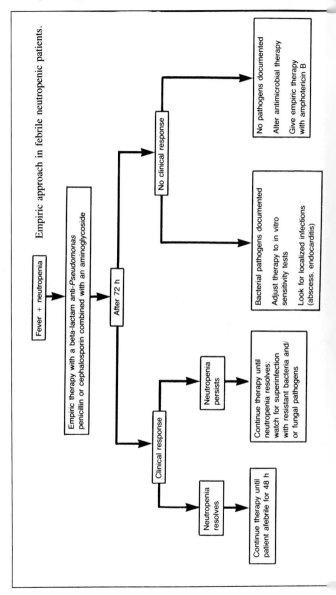

Empiric approach in febrile neutropenic patients.

Stage-specific diagnostic approach to FUO

Stage 1: Screening (in all adult patients with FUO)

    History: Specific symptoms; review of systems; immunization; travel; animal exposure; medications and drugs; sex; work; recreation

    Physical examination: Fever documentation, general examination with special attention to skin, lymphnodes, fundi, heart and lungs, abdomen, joints

    Hematology: Complete blood count and differential, ESR

    Chemistry: Liver function tests, protein electrophoresis

    Urine analysis: Cells; chemistry

    Cultures: Blood (aerob and anaerob, mycobacteria, fungi, viruses); urine; CSF and other body fluids, if obtained

    Serologies: Brucellosis, syphilis, Lyme, HIV, CMV, EBV, amebiasis, toxoplasmosis, chlamydia; ANA, rheumatoid factors, antistreptolysin-O

    Imaging: Regular chest radiogram; abdominal ultrasound

    Others: Skin tests (PPD and control); ECG; bone marrow aspirate (?)

Stage 2: Noninvasive approach to suspected diagnoses

    CT scan: Abdomen (intraabdominal tumors or abscesses; liver abscesses); chest (lung tumors); head (lymphoma, toxoplasmosis, abscess)

    Radiograms: Intravenous pyelogram (urinary tract abnormalities); bone films (osteomyelitis); retrograde cholangiography (cholangitis)

    Endoscopies: GI-tract (Crohn's disease); bronchial tree (bronchus tumors)

    Radionucleotide studies: Bone (osteomyelitis); thyroid gland (thyreoiditis); pulmonary perfusion/ventilation (emboli)

    Echocardiogram: (Cardiac tumors, endocarditis)

Stage 3: Invasive approach to suspected diagnosis

    Biopsies: Lymph nodes, tumors, skin lesions, liver, bone marrow

    Laparascopy (if evidence for intra-abdominal process obtained during stage 1 or 2)

Stage 4: Failure to establish a diagnosis

    Reevaluate patient at regular intervals (if clinical status not rapidly deteriorating)

    Empiric therapy: Nonsteroidal anti-inflammatory drugs; corticosteroids; antituberculous drugs; antibiotics

ESR, erythrocyte sedimentation rate, CMV, cytomegalovirus, EBV, Epstein-Barr virus.

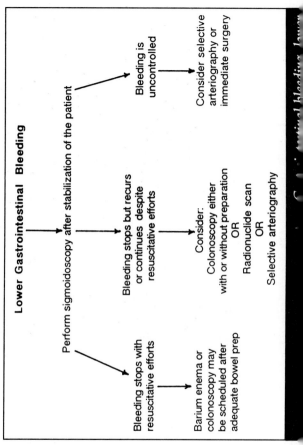

Scheme for the diagnostic evaluation of acute lower gastrointestinal bleeding.

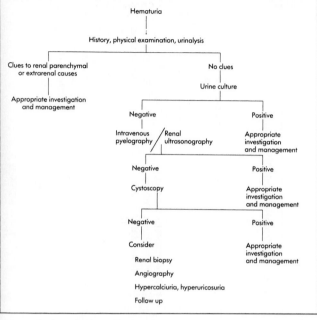

Strategy for investigation of hematuria

DIAGNOSTIC APPROACH TO HYPERNATREMIA

CLINICALLY ASSESS EXTRACELLULAR FLUID VOLUME

DEPLETED / NORMAL / EXPANDED

HYPOVOLEMIC HYPERNATREMIA
LOSS OF WATER+Na (H_2O LOSS > Na)

CAUSES	BUN/Cr	URINARY (Na)	Osm
RENAL:			
DIURETICS	↑/↑	↓	↓
GLYCOSURIA	↑/N↑	↑	↓
UREA DIURESIS	↑/N↑	↑	↓
ACUTE/CHRONIC RENAL FAIL.	↑/↑↑	↑	↓
PARTIAL OBST.			
ADRENAL:			
CONG./ACQ. DEFICIENCIES	↑↑/↑	↑	↑↑
GI LOSSES	↑↑/↑	↓	↑
RESPIRATORY LOSSES	↑↑/↑	↓	↑
SKIN LOSSES	↑↑/↑	↓	↑

ISOVOLEMIC HYPERNATREMIA
LOSS OF WATER

CAUSES	BUN/Cr	URINARY (Na)	Osm
DIABET. INSIP.			
CENTRAL	↑/N	N	↓
NEPHROG.	↑/N	N	↓
RESET			
OSMOSTAT	N/N	↑	V
SKIN LOSS	↑/N	↓	↑
IATROGENIC	N/N	V	↓

HYPERVOLEMIC HYPERNATREMIA
GAIN WATER+Na (Na GAIN > H_2O)

CAUSES	BUN/Cr	URINARY (Na)	Osm
IATROGENIC	V	↑(↓V)	V
MINERALOCORT. EXCESS			
1° ALDO	N	N	↑
CUSHING'S	N	N	↑
CONG. ADR. HYPERPLAS.	N	N	↑
EXOGENOUS	N	N	↑

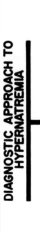

Differential diagnosis of hypernatremia: the clinical and laboratory approach to the classification and diagnosis of the hypernatremic disorders is illustrated. N, normal; V, variable; INSP, insipidus. (From Narins RG et al: Diagnostic strategies in disorders of fluid, electrolyte, and acid-base homeostasis, Am J Med 72:496, 1982.)

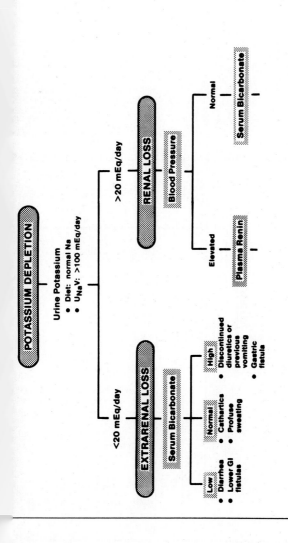

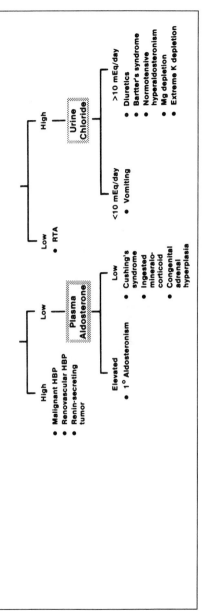

Diagnostic approach to hypokalemia. Because renal potassium wasting may improve during sodium restriction, diminished potassium excretion is indicative of extrarenal loss only when the diet (and therefore the urine) is rich in sodium.

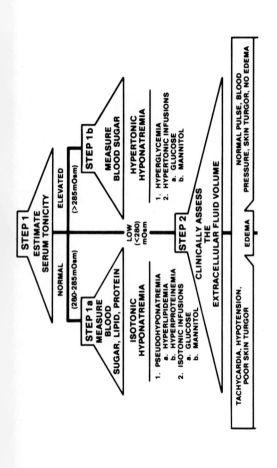

STEP 1
ESTIMATE
SERUM TONICITY

NORMAL
(280-285mOsm)

ELEVATED
(>285mOsm)

LOW
(<280)
mOsm

STEP 1a
MEASURE
BLOOD
SUGAR, LIPID, PROTEIN

ISOTONIC
HYPONATREMIA

1. PSEUDOHYPONATREMIA
   a. HYPERLIPIDEMIA
   b. HYPERPROTEINEMIA
2. ISOTONIC INFUSIONS
   a. GLUCOSE
   b. MANNITOL

STEP 1b
MEASURE
BLOOD SUGAR

HYPERTONIC
HYPONATREMIA

1. HYPERGLYCEMIA
2. HYPERTONIC INFUSIONS
   a. GLUCOSE
   b. MANNITOL

STEP 2
CLINICALLY ASSESS
THE
EXTRACELLULAR FLUID VOLUME

TACHYCARDIA, HYPOTENSION,
POOR SKIN TURGOR

EDEMA

NORMAL PULSE, BLOOD
PRESSURE, SKIN TURGOR, NO EDEMA

I. HYPOVOLEMIC HYPOTONIC HYPONATREMIA

CAUSES	BUN/Cr	URIC ACID	URINARY Osm.	Na
1. GI LOSSES	↑↑/↑	↑	↑↑	↓↓
2. SKIN LOSSES	↑↑/↑	↑	↑↑	↓↓
3. LUNG LOSSES	↑↑/↑	↑	↑↑	↓↓
4. 3rd SPACE	↑↑/↑	↑	↑↑	↓↓
5. RENAL LOSSES				
a. DIURETICS	↑↑/↑	↑	ISO	↑
b. RENAL DAMAGE	↑↑/↑↑	↑	ISO	↑
c. PARTIAL URINARY TRACT OBSTRUCT.	↑↑/↑	↑	ISO	(↑)
6. ADRENAL INSUFFICIENCY	↑↑/↑	↑	↑	↑

II. HYPERVOLEMIC HYPOTONIC HYPONATREMIA

CAUSES	BUN/Cr	URIC ACID	URINARY Osm.	Na
1. CHF	↑↑/↑	↑	↑	↓
2. LIVER DAMAGE	↑↑/↑	↑	↑	↓
3. NEPHROSIS	↑↑/↑ (↑↑/↑↑)	↑	(ISO ↑)	↓

III. ISOVOLEMIC HYPOTONIC HYPONATREMIA

CAUSES	BUN/Cr	URIC ACID	URINARY Osm.	Na
1. H_2O INTOX	↓/↓	↓	↓(↓)	↓
2. RENAL FAIL.	↑↑/↑↑	↑	ISO	ISO
3. K+ LOSS	↑/↑(N)	↑	↑	↑
4. SIADH	↓/↓	↓↓	↑	↑
5. RESET OSMOSTAT	N	N	V	V

Differential diagnosis of hyponatremia. The figure integrates the classification of the hyponatremias with a clinical and laboratory approach to their diagnosis. CHF, congestive heart failure; ISO, isotonic; N, normal; V, variable. (Modified from Narins RG et al: Diagnostic strategies in disorders of fluid, electrolyte, and acid-base homeostasis, Am J Med 72:496, 1982.)

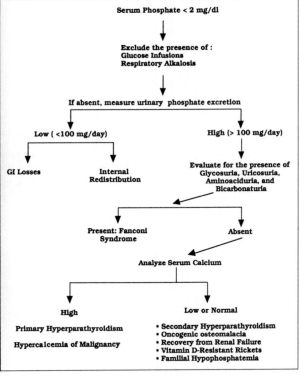

Diagnostic work-up of hypophosphatemia.

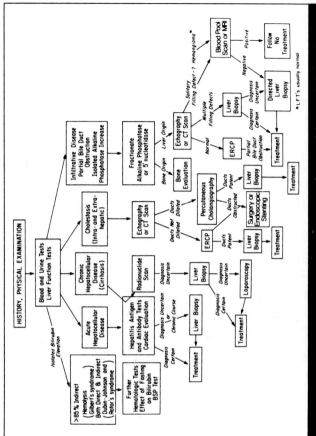

Evaluation of jaundice and hepatobiliary disease. *BSP*, Bromsulphalein; *CT*, computed tomography; *ERCP*, endoscopic retrograde cholangiopancreatography; *LFTs*, liver function tests.

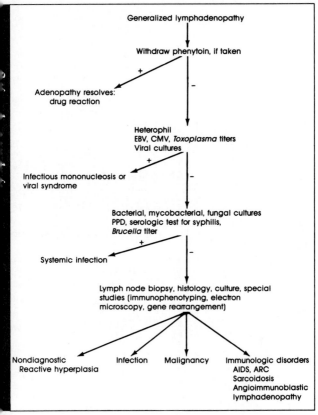

Clinical approach to the patient with generalized lymphadenopathy.

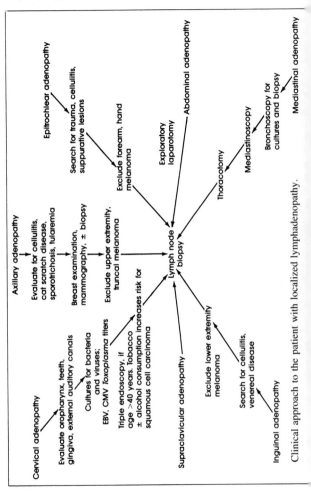

Clinical approach to the patient with localized lymphadenopathy.

Cervical adenopathy
Evaluate oropharynx, teeth, gingiva, external auditory canals
Cultures for bacteria and viruses; EBV, CMV *Toxoplasma* titers
Triple endoscopy, If age >40 years. Tobacco ± alcohol consumption increases risk for squamous cell carcinoma

Axillary adenopathy
Evaluate for cellulitis, cat scratch disease, sporotrichosis, tularemia
Breast examination, mammography, ± biopsy
Exclude upper extremity, truncal melanoma

Epitrochlear adenopathy
Search for trauma, cellulitis, suppurative lesions
Exclude forearm, hand melanoma

Abdominal adenopathy
Exploratory laparotomy

Mediastinal adenopathy
Bronchoscopy for cultures and biopsy
Mediastinoscopy
Thoracotomy

Lymph node biopsy

Supraclavicular adenopathy
Exclude lower extremity melanoma

Inguinal adenopathy
Search for cellulitis, venereal disease

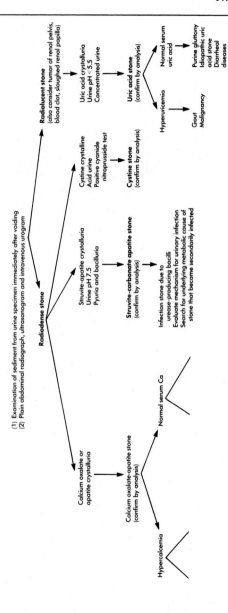

(1) Examination of sediment from urine specimen immediately after voiding
(2) Plain abdominal radiograph, ultrasonogram and intravenous urogram

Radiolucent stone
(also consider tumor of renal pelvis, blood clot, sloughed renal papilla)

Uric acid crystalluria
Urine pH < 5.5
Concentrated urine

Uric acid stone
(confirm by analysis)

Hyperuricemia

Gout
Malignancy

Normal serum uric acid

Purine gluttony
Idiopathic uric acid stone
Diarrheal diseases

Radiodense stone

Cystine crystalline
Acid urine
Positive cyanide nitroprusside test

Cystine stone
(confirm by analysis)

Struvite-apatite crystalluria
Urine pH 7.5
Pyuria and bacilluria

Struvite-carbonate apatite stone
(confirm by analysis)

Infection stone due to urease-producing bacilli
Evaluate mechanism for urinary infection
Search for underlying metabolic cause of stone that became secondarily infected

Calcium oxalate or apatite crystalluria

Calcium oxalate-apatite stone
(confirm by analysis)

Normal serum Ca

Hypercalcemia

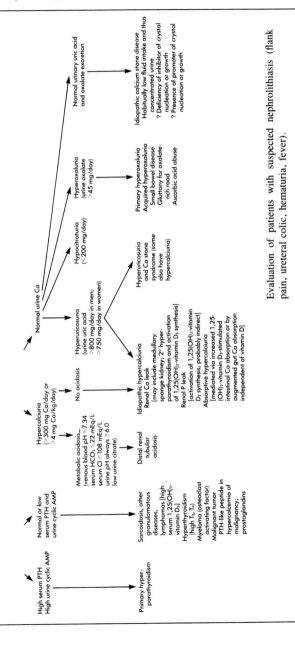

Evaluation of patients with suspected nephrolithiasis (flank pain, ureteral colic, hematuria, fever).

High serum PTH
High urine cyclic AMP

Primary hyperparathyroidism

Normal or low serum PTH and urine cyclic AMP

Sarcoidosis, other granulomatous diseases, lymphomas [high serum 1,25(OH)$_2$-vitamin D$_3$]
Hyperthyroidism (high T$_4$, T$_3$)
Myeloma (osteoclast activating factor)
Malignant tumor PTH-like peptide in hypercalcemia of malignancy; prostaglandins

Hypercalciuria (>300 mg Ca/day or >4 mg Ca/kg/day)

Metabolic acidosis—(venous blood pH ≤7.34 serum HCO$_3$ ≤22 mEq/L serum Cl ≥108 mEq/L urine pH always ≥6.0 low urine citrate)

Distal renal tubular acidosis

No acidosis

Idiopathic hypercalciuria
Renal Ca leak [may include medullary sponge kidney; 2° hyperparathyroidism and activation of 1,25(OH)$_2$-vitamin D$_3$ synthesis]
Renal P leak [activation of 1,25(OH)$_2$-vitamin D$_3$ synthesis; probably indirect]
Absorptive hypercalciuria [mediated via increased 1,25-(OH)$_2$-vitamin D$_3$-stimulated intestinal Ca absorption or by augmented gut Ca absorption independent of vitamin D]

Normal urine Ca

Hyperuricosuria (urine uric acid >800 mg/day in men; >750 mg/day in women)

Hyperuricosuria and Ca stone syndrome (some also have hypercalciuria)

Hypocitraturia (<200 mg/day)

Hyperoxaluria (urine oxalate >45 mg/day)

Primary hyperoxaluria
Acquired hyperoxaluria
Small bowel disease
Gluttony for oxalate-rich road
Ascorbic acid abuse

Normal urinary uric acid and oxalate excretion

Idiopathic calcium stone disease
Habitually low fluid intake and thus concentrated urine
? Deficiency of inhibitor of crystal nucleation or growth
? Presence of promoter of crystal nucleation or growth

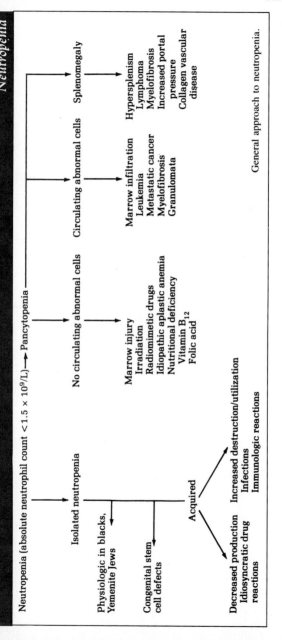

Neutropenia

Neutropenia (absolute neutrophil count $<1.5 \times 10^9/L$) ⟶ Pancytopenia

Isolated neutropenia

Physiologic in blacks,
Yemenite Jews

Congenital stem
cell defects

Acquired

Decreased production
Idiosyncratic drug
reactions

Increased destruction/utilization
Infections
Immunologic reactions

No circulating abnormal cells

Marrow injury
Irradiation
Radiomimetic drugs
Idiopathic aplastic anemia
Nutritional deficiency
Vitamin B₁₂
Folic acid

Circulating abnormal cells

Marrow infiltration
Leukemia
Metastatic cancer
Myelofibrosis
Granulomata

Splenomegaly

Hypersplenism
Lymphoma
Myelofibrosis
Increased portal
pressure
Collagen vascular
disease

General approach to neutropenia.

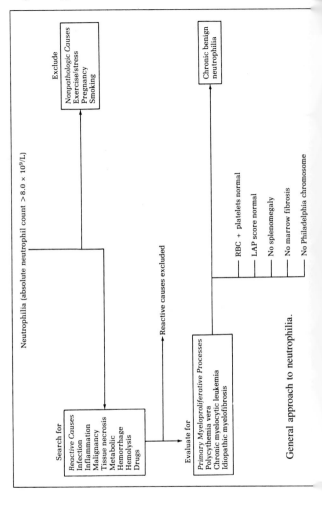

Neutrophilia (absolute neutrophil count >8.0 × 10⁹/L)

Exclude

Nonpathologic Causes
Exercise/stress
Pregnancy
Smoking

Search for

Reactive Causes
Infection
Inflammation
Malignancy
Tissue necrosis
Metabolic
Hemorrhage
Hemolysis
Drugs

Reactive causes excluded

Evaluate for

Primary Myeloproliferative Processes
Polycythemia vera
Chronic myelocytic leukemia
Idiopathic myelofibrosis

Chronic benign neutrophilia

RBC + platelets normal
LAP score normal
No splenomegaly
No marrow fibrosis
No Philadelphia chromosome

General approach to neutrophilia.

Information useful for the diagnosis of pleural effusions

I. Specific diagnostic aids
   A. Positive smear and/or culture for bacteria, mycobacteria, or fungi
   B. Positive cytology for primary or metastatic neoplasm or for lymphoma
   C. "True" chylous effusion-disruption or invasion of thoracic ducts
II. Potentially useful characteristics in differential diagnosis
   A. Elevated pleural fluid amylase/serum amylase ratio suggests
      1. Pancreatitis
      2. Pancreatic pseudocyst
      3. Ruptured esophagus (salivary amylase)
      4. Neoplasm
   B. Pleural fluid/serum glucose ratio <0.5 suggests tuberculosis, tumor, parapneumonic effusion, rheumatoid arthritis, or systemic lupus erythematosus
   C. Red blood count >100,000/mm^3 associated most often with tumors, trauma, and embolus with infarction
   D. Lymphocytosis in exudate (>50% lymphocytes) seen in chronic effusions
   E. Pleural fluid eosinophilia rare in malignant and tuberculous effusions unless there is a coincident pneumothorax
   F. Greater than 1% mesothelial cells rare in tuberculous effusion
   G. Pseudochylous effusions (cholesterol crystals) seen with chronic effusion of rheumatoid disease, tuberculosis, and trapped lung
   H. Elevated acid mucopolysaccharide and hyaluronic acid levels usually associated with mesothelioma
   I. Lupus erythematosus cells: presence diagnostic of lupus pleuritis
   J. pH <7.1 in parapneumonic effusion suggests, but alone does not mandate, need for closed-tube thoracostomy
   K. Foul-smelling odor characteristic of anaerobic infection

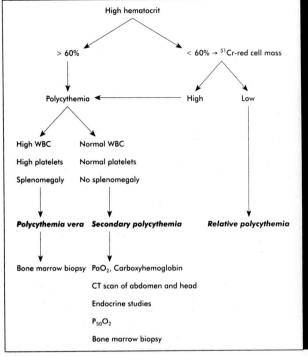

Evaluation of a patient with a high hematocrit.

Diagnostic evaluation of the patient with Raynaud's phenomenon

History: including occupational and drug exposure, smoking, symptoms of connective tissue disease, frequency and duration of RP attacks

Physical examination: including skin examination, palpation of peripheral pulses, auscultation for bruits

Laboratory studies: complete blood count, ESR, thyroid function tests, cryoglobulins, ANA, nailfold capillary microscopy

Ancillary tests: anticentromere, anti-Scl-70 and anti-DNA antibodies if screening ANA positive or connective tissue disease suspected; arteriography only if peripheral pulses asymmetric or diminished

Modified from Maricq HR et al: Diagnostic potential of in vivo capillary microscopy in scleroderma and related disorders. Arthritis Rheum 23:183, 1980.

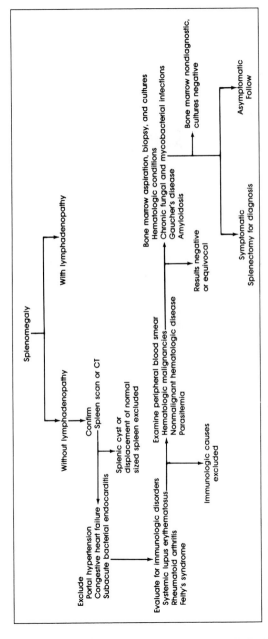

Clinical approach to the patient with splenomegaly.

Questions to ask the patient and observers in the evaluation of syncope

Questions for the patient

1. What were you doing during the hours and minutes preceding the blackout?
2. What was your situation regarding loss of sleep, ingestion of food and alcohol, and use of drugs or medications prior to the black-out?
3. What was your body position or posture?
4. What was the first thing you noticed to be wrong?
5. What symptoms did you experience next, in what order, and for how long?
6. Do you remember slumping or striking the floor?
7. What was the next thing you remember, and what position were you in when you regained awareness?
8. Did you hurt yourself in the fall?
   a. Did you injure your tongue or mouth?
   b. Did your back or muscles ache?
   c. Did you have a headache?
   d. Did you lose control of your bladder or bowels?
   e. How did you feel on awakening, and how long did it take for you to feel entirely normal again—seconds, minutes, or longer?

Questions for the observers

1. Ask the observers to answer the preceding questions when appropriate.
2. Was there any turning of the eyes or head?
3. Was there any twitching or jerking of the face or extremities?
4. Was the skin sweaty, pale, flushed, or blue?
5. Did the patient respond to observers in any way during the apparent unconsciousness?

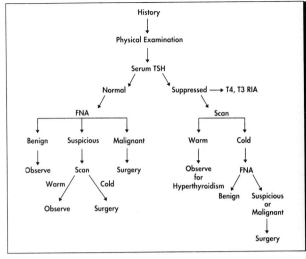

Evaluation of a patient with a palpable thyroid nodule.

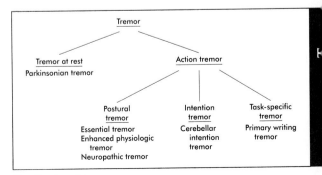

Classification of tremor.

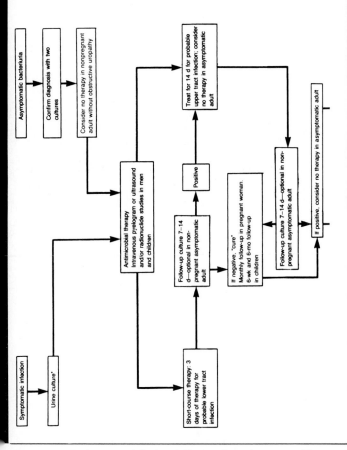

Management of urinary tract infections.* Not mandatory in women with only lower tract symptoms.

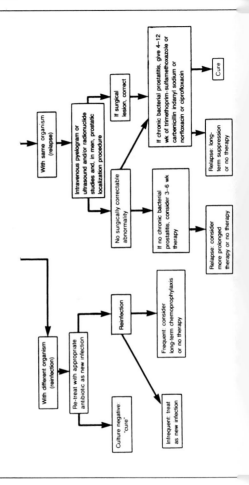

Therapeutic Modalities

Empiric antimicrobial regimens for suspected anaerobic or mixed infections

Site	Treatment of choice	Alternate regimens
Pleuropulmonary, odontogenic, or human bite infections	Penicillin G IV, 1-4 MU q4h or ampicillin-sulbactam IV, 1-2 g q6h	Clindamycin IV, 600 mg q6h Cefoxitin IV, 1-2 g q6h Cefotaxime IV, 2 g q6h
Brain abscess or subdural empyema	Penicillin G IV, 4 MU q4h + metronidazole IV, 500 mg q6h	Penicillin G IV, 4 MU q4h + chloramphenicol 500 mg q6h
Intra-abdominal, pelvic, or necrotic soft tissue infections	Clindamycin IV, 600 mg q6h or metronidazole IV, 500 mg q6h; each + tobramycin IV, q8h or ciprofloxacin IV, 200 mg q12h	Cefoxitin IV, 2 g q6h, cefotetan IV, 2 g q12h, ceftizoxime IV, 3 g q8h, piperacillin IV, 3 g q4h, imipenem IV, 500 mg q6h, or piperacillin-tazobactam IV, 2-4 g q4-6h; each ± tobramycin IV, q8h or ciprofloxacin IV, q12h

Antibiotic use during pregnancy

Antibiotic	Special considerations during pregnancy
Penicillin G	Safe in nonallergic patients; dosage requirements increased during pregnancy
Ampicillin	Dosage requirements increased during pregnancy; can lower urinary estriols; unconjugated serum estriol unaffected
Amoxicillin	Same as ampicillin
Oxacillin	Dosage requirements increased during pregnancy
Cephalosporins	Dosage requirements increased during pregnancy; some cross-sensitivity in penicillin-allergic patients; may affect urinary estriols; no effect on unconjugated serum estriol
Erythromycin	Generally safe; placental transfer is erratic, but the fetal liver concentrates the drug
Tetracycline	Abnormal fetal teeth and bone development; increased risk of maternal liver and pancreatic disease; contraindicated in pregnancy
Chloramphenicol	May cause "gray baby syndrome"; avoid in pregnancy
Clindamycin	Fetal effects are unknown; may rarely cause pseudomembranous colitis in the mother
Vancomycin	Potential fetal ototoxicity; should be reserved for life-threatening infections in patients allergic to penicillin
Metronidazole	Mutagenic and carcinogenic in animals; may be necessary to use for symptomatic parasitic infections during second and third trimesters
Nitrofurantoin	Generally safe but has been rarely associated with hemolytic anemia in the newborn; few systemic effects
Quinolones	Contraindicated in pregnancy
Sulfonamides	Competes with bilirubin for albumin binding; should not be used in last trimester to avoid neonatal kernicterus
Trimethoprim	Folic acid antagonist; should be avoided during pregnancy unless no alternative available
Aminoglycosides Amikacin Gentamicin Kanamycin Streptomycin Tobramycin	Possible fetal and maternal ototoxicity and renal toxicity; maternal serum levels should be monitored closely but are usually in low range because of rapid renal clearance

Concomitant diseases and the choice of antihypertensive drug therapy

	Indications	Contraindications
Diuretics	Congestive heart failure Volume retention	Diabetes Gout Hypercholesterolemia
Central alpha agonists	Withdrawal from addictive behaviors (clonidine)	Liver disease (methyldopa) Autoimmune disease (methyldopa) Depression
Alpha blockers	Hypercholesterolemia High level of physical activity	Postural hypotension
Beta blockers	Coronary artery disease Tachyarrhythmias Migraine Anxiety	Asthma Diabetes requiring insulin Bradyarrhythmias Congestive heart failure Peripheral vascular disease Hypertriglyceridemia
ACE inhibitors	Congestive heart failure Renal insufficiency Peripheral vascular disease	Renal failure Renovascular hypertension Volume depletion Pregnancy
Calcium antagonists	Coronary artery disease Tachyarrhythmias (verapamil) Peripheral vascular disease	Bradyarrhythmias (verapamil)

Antihypertensives and concomitant diseases

Antimicrobial drugs of choice*

Infecting organism	Antimicrobial of choice
Gram-positive cocci	
S. aureus or *epidermidis*	
Non-penicillinase-producing	Penicillin G or V
Penicillinase-producing	Penicillinase-resistant penicillin‡
Methicillin-resistant	Vancomycin (± gentamicin and/or rifampin)
Beta streptococci (groups A, B, C, G)	Penicillin G or V
Streptococcus, viridans group	Penicillin G
Streptococcus bovis	Penicillin G
Enterococci	
Uncomplicated urinary tract infection	Ampicillin or amoxicillin
Endocarditis or other serious infection	Penicillin G (or ampicillin) plus gentamicin or streptomycin
Pneumococcus	Penicillin G or V
Gram-negative cocci	
N. gonorrhoeae	Ceftriaxone
N. meningitidis	Penicillin G

Alternative drugs

Cephalosporin,† vancomycin, clindamycin, erythromycin
Cephalosporin,† vancomycin, clindamycin, erythromycin, imipenem
Trimethoprim-sulfamethoxazole, monocycline

Erythromycin, cephalosporin,† vancomycin

Cephalosporin,† vancomycin, erythromycin
Cephalosporin,† vancomycin, erythromycin

Nitrofurantoin, quinolone§

Vancomycin plus gentamicin or streptomycin

Erythromycin, cephalosporin,† chloramphenicol, vancomycin

Ampicillin, amoxicillin, penicillin G, spectinomycin, cefoxitin, cefuroxime,
    cefotaxime, ceftizoxime, quinolone,§ erythromycin
Chloramphenicol, cefuroxime, ceftriaxone, ceftizoxime, cefotaxime, sulfonamide,
    trimethoprim-sulfamethoxazole

Continued.

Antimicrobial drugs of choice—cont'd

Infecting organism	Antimicrobial of choice
Gram-positive bacilli	
Bacillus anthracis (anthrax)	Penicillin G
Corynebacterium diphtheriae	Erythromycin
Listeria monocytogenes	Ampicillin or penicillin G (± gentamicin)
Gram-negative bacilli	
Acinetobacter sp.	Imipenem
Bordetella pertussis (whooping cough)	Erythromycin
Brucella sp. (brucellosis)	Tetracycline (± streptomycin)
Campylobacter jejuni	Erythromycin
Enterobacter sp.	Aminoglycoside,‖ imipenem broad spectrum penicillin,** trimethoprim-sulfamethoxazole
E. coli	
Uncomplicated urinary tract infection	Trimethoprim-sulfamethoxazole or amoxicillin clavulanate
Systemic infection	Aminoglycoside‖ or cephalosporin†
Francisella tularensis (tularemia)	Streptomycin
H. influenzae	
Meningitis, epiglottitis, bacteremia	Ceftriaxone, cefotaxime, or ceftizoxime
Other infections	Ampicillin or amoxicillin, ampicillin-sulbactam, amoxicillin-clavulanate
Klebsiella pneumoniae	Aminoglycoside‖ (for serious infections, cefotaxime, ceftizoxime, ceftazidime, or ceftriaxone)
Legionella pneumophila	Erythromycin
Pasteurella multocida	Penicillin G
Proteus mirabilis	Ampicillin

Alternative drugs

Erythromycin, tetracyline
Penicillin G
Trimethoprim-sulfamethoxazole, chloramphenicol, tetracycline, erythromycin

Aminoglycoside,‖ broad spectrum penicillin, trimethoprim-sulfamethoxazole, doxycycline
Trimethoprim-sulfamethoxazole, ampicillin

Chloramphenicol (± streptomycin)
Tetracycline, gentamicin, quinolone§
Quinolone§, cefotaxime, ceftizoxime, ceftriaxone, chloramphenicol, tetracycline

Cephalosporin,† tetracycline, ampicillin, amoxicillin, trimethoprim, quinolone§

Ampicillin,† broad-spectrum penicillin,** trimethoprim-sulfamethoxazole, chloramphenicol, ampicillin-sulbactam, ticarcillin-clavulanate
Tetracycline, chloramphenicol

Trimethoprim-sulfamethoxazole, ampicillin plus chloramphenicol initially

Trimethoprim-sulfamethoxazole, cefamandole, cefixime, cefprozil, cefuroxime, cefonicid, cefaclor, ceftriaxone, cefotaxime, ceftizoxime, sulfonamide, tetracycline, quinolone†
Cephalosporin† (for serious infections, cefotaxime, ceftizoxime, ceftazidime, or ceftriaxone), ampicillin-sulbactam, trimethoprim-sulfamethoxazole, quinolone†, extended spectrum penicillin, chloramphenicol, tetracycline, ticarcillin-clavulanate
Add rifampin, quinolone
Tetracycline, cephalosporin,† amoxicillin-clavulanate
Cephalosporin,† aminoglycoside,‖ broad spectrum penicillin,** trimethoprim-sulfamethoxazole, chloramphenicol, quinolone†

Continued

Antimicrobial drugs of choice—cont'd

Infecting organism	Antimicrobial of choice
Gram-negative bacilli—cont'd	
Proteus, indole-positive	Aminoglycoside‖
Pseudomonas aeruginosa	
Urinary infection	Broad spectrum penicillin,** quinolone†
Other infection	Aminoglycoside‖ ± broad spectrum penicillin**
Salmonella sp.	Quinolone† or ceftriaxone or cefotaxime
Serratia marcescens	Aminoglycoside‖ or cefotaxime, ceftazidime, ceftizoxime
Shigella sp.	Quinolone§
Yersinia pestis (plague)	Streptomycin
Anaerobes	
Anaerobic streptococci	Penicillin G
Bacteroides sp.	
Oropharyngeal strains	Penicillin G
Gastrointestinal strains	Clindamycin or metronidazole
Clostridium sp.	Penicillin G

*Not all drugs listed are approved for that indication by the US Food and Drug Administration.

†A first-generation cephalosporin (cephalothin, cephapirin, cefazolin, cephradine, cephalexin, cefadroxil, cefaclor) is preferred. Enteric gram-negative bacilli resistant to these agents may be susceptible to second or third generation cephalosporins.

‡Methicillin, nafcillin, oxacillin, cloxacillin, dicloxacillin.

‖Gentamicin, tobramycin, netilmicin, amikacin.

**Carbenicillin, ticarcillin, mezlocillin, piperacillin, azlocillin.

§Ciprofloxacin, Lomefloxacin, Ofloxacin or (for urinary tract infections only) norfloxacin, enoxacin.

Alternative drugs

Cefotaxime, ceftizoxime, ceftriaxone, ceftazidime, ticarcillin-clavulanate, broad
  spectrum penicillin,** trimethoprim-sulfamethoxazole, chloramphenicol, tetracycline, quinolone,§ imipenem

Aminoglycoside,‖ ceftazidime, imipenem

Ceftazidime ± aminoglycoside, imipenem ± aminoglycoside, ciproflaxacin

Ampicillin, amoxicillin, chloramphenicol, trimethoprim-sulfamethoxazole

Trimethoprim-sulfamethoxazole, broad spectrum penicillin,** chloramphenicol,
  quinolone,† imipenem
Trimethoprim-sulfamethoxazole, ampicillin, chloramphenicol, tetracycline
Tetracycline, chloramphenicol

Clindamycin, chloramphenicol, cephalosporin,† erythromycin

Clindamycin, cefoxitin, chloramphenicol, metronidazole, cefotetan, cefmetazole,
  imipenem, ampicillin-sulbactam, ticarcillin-clavulanate
Cefoxitin, chloramphenicol, cefotetan, cefmetazole, imipenem, ampicillin-
  sulbactam, ticarcillin-clavulanate
Chloramphenicol, clindamycin, metronidazole

Treatment of candidiasis

Form of disease	Treatment regimen	Comments
Uncomplicated mucosal disease	For thrush, clotrimazole troches or nystatin. For esophagitis, ketoconazole or fluconazole. For intertriginous disease or vaginal disease, topical miconazole, clotrimazole.	Fluconazole and ketoconazole are effective but should be reserved for severe or refractory infections. In AIDS patients, fluconazole has been more effective than ketoconazole.
Chronic mucocutaneous candidiasis	Ketoconazole 200 to 600 mg/day, P.O. Fluconazole 200 mg/day, P.O.	For control, intermittent I.V. amphotericin B may be necessary.
Upper urinary tract infection	Intravenous amphotericin B, 0.3–0.6 mg/kg/day until evidence of resolution. Fluconazole is under investigation.	
Cystitis	Remove catheter, amphotericin B bladder washout. 5-FC, 50–75 mg/kg/day, P.O. Fluconazole under investigation. For severe cases, amphotericin B, I.V.	Resistance to 5-FC may be present and also may develop during therapy.
Disseminated candidiasis and candidemia	Amphotericin B, 0.3–0.6 mg/kg/day for 1 to 3 weeks depending on severity. Flucytosine, 100 to 150 mg/kg/day, P.O., may be added depending on severity. Patients with catheter-associated candidemia and a low probability of having disseminated candidiasis should receive fluconazole, 200 to 400 mg/day. All patients with candidemia, whether or not it is associated with a catheter, should be treated with an antifungal unless there is a contraindication.	A large, multicenter clinical trial comparing amphotericin B with fluconazole in candidemia is in progress. It will clarify the role of fluconazole when completed.

Candida endophthalmitis	Amphotericin B at 0.3 to 0.6 mg/kg/day until evidence of resolution occurs. In severe cases or in cases where the macula is involved, 5-FC, 100-150 mg/kg/day, P.O., should be added. Fluconazole is under investigation.	Partial vitrectomy should be considered with ophthalmological consultation.
Candida endocarditis	Infected valve should be removed as soon as possible. After surgery, amphotericin B and 5-FC should be given for 6 weeks or more.	There are reports of rare cases of cure with amphotericin B therapy. They are the exception and the valve should be removed whenever possible.
Prosthetic implants infected with *Candida*	Removal of implant is almost always necessary. Amphotericin B should be given after removal.	The role of fluconazole is not yet known.

Current recommendations for treatment of bacterial endocarditis

Antibiotics	Dosage[a]	Administration	Duration	Comments
Penicillin-susceptible viridans streptococci and *Streptococcus bovis* (MIC ≤ 0.1 µg/ml)				
1. Penicillin G	2 million units every 4 hr	IV	4 wk	Preferred in patients >65 years old and those with renal or eight cranial nerve impairment, heart failure, or CNS complications. Effective for other penicillin-susceptible nonviridans streptococci.
2. Penicillin G & gentamicin[b]	2 million units every 4 hr 1 mg/kg (not to exceed 80 mg) q8h	IV IV	2 wk 2 wk	Uncomplicated patient: age <65; no renal or eight cranial nerve impairment; no CNS complication; no severe heart failure; not nutritionally deficient variant; viridans streptococci and *S. bovis* only.
3. Penicillin G & gentamicin[b]	2 million units every 4 hr 1 mg/kg (not to exceed 80 mg) q8h	IV IV	4 wk 2 wk	Nutritionally deficient variants; relapse; complications such as shock or extra-cardiac focus of infection; 6 wks of penicillin for prosthetic valve infection.
4. Vancomycin[c]	15 mg/kg (not to exceed 1 g) q12h	IV	4 wk	Penicillin allergy.
5. Cefazolin[d]	1-2 g every 8 hr	IV	4 wk	Penicillin allergy.
6. Ceftriaxone[d]	2 g once daily	IV or IM	4 wk	Uncomplicated patient with viridans streptococci; candidate for outpatient therapy; penicillin allergy.

Strains of viridans streptococci & S. *bovis* relatively resistant to penicillin G (0.1 µg/ml < MIC < 0.5 µg/ml)

1. Penicillin G	2 million units every 4 hr	IV	4 wk	For MIC >0.5 µg/ml, treat same as enterococcus. For prosthetic valve infection, give 6 wk of penicillin and 6 wk of gentamicin.
& gentamicin[b]	1 mg/kg (not to exceed 80 mg) q8h	IV	2 wk	
2. Vancomycin[c]	15 mg/kg (not to exceed 1 g) q12h	IV	4 wk	Penicillin allergy; avoidance of gentamicin.
3. Cefazolin[d]	1-2 g every 8 hr	IV	4 wk	Penicillin allergy; avoidance of gentamicin.

Enterococci (E. *faecalis*) (or viridans streptococci with MIC ≥0.5 µg/ml)

1. Penicillin G	4 million units every 4 hr	IV	4-6 wk	Increase to 6-8 wks for symptoms longer than 3 months, complicated course, or prosthetic valve infection. Some would use ampicillin, but no evidence of superiority available.
& gentamicin[b]	1 mg/kg (not to exceed 80 mg) q8h	IV	4-6 wk	
2. Vancomycin[c]	15 mg/kg (not to exceed 1 g) q12h	IV	4-6 wk	Penicillin allergy.
& gentamicin[b]	1 mg/kg (not to exceed 80 mg) q8h	IV	4-6 wk	

Continued.

Current recommendations for treatment of bacterial endocarditis—cont'd

Antibiotics	Dosage[a]	Administration	Duration	Comments
Staphylococcus aureus				
1. Nafcillin	1.5 g every 4 hr	IV	4 wk	Methicillin-susceptible strain; increase duration to 6 wks for complicated infection; omit gentamicin for significant renal impairment. Some recommend gentamicin for 5-7 days.
& gentamicin[b]	1 mg/kg (not to exceed 80 mg) q8h	IV	3-5 days	
2. Vancomycin[c]	15 mg/kg (not to exceed 1 g) q12h	IV	4-6 wk	Penicillin allergy or methicillin-resistant strain; increase duration to 6 wks or longer for complicated infection.
3. Cefazolin[d]	2 g every 8 hr	IV	4-6 wk	Penicillin allergy; increase duration to 6 wks for complicated infection.
4. Nafcillin	1.5 g every 4 hr	IV	2 wk	Methicillin-susceptible strain; intravenous drug user, tricuspid valve infection only, no extrapulmonary infection, no renal impairment.
& gentamicin[b]	1 mg/kg (not to exceed 80 mg) q8h	IV	2 wk	
5. Nafcillin	1.5 g every 4 hr	IV	6-8 wk	Prosthetic valve infected with methicillin-susceptible strain; for methicillin-resistant strain substitute vancomycin for nafcillin.
& rifampin[e]	300 mg every 12 hr	PO or IV	6 wk	
& gentamicin[b]	1 mg/kg (not to exceed 80 mg) q8h	IV	2 wk	

Coagulase-negative staphylococci or prosthetic valve infection

1. Nafcillin	1.5 g every 4 hr	IV	6-8 wk	Methicillin-susceptible strain; vancomycin recommended in case of uncertain methicillin susceptibility.
& rifampin	300 mg every 12 hr	PO or IV	6-8 wk	
& gentamicin[b]	1 mg/kg (not to exceed 80 mg) q8h	IV	2 wk	
2. Vancomycin[c]	15 mg/kg (not to exceed 1 g) q12h	IV	6-8 wk	Methicillin-resistant strain; penicillin allergy.
& rifampin	300 mg every 12 hr	PO or IV	6-8 wk	
& gentamicin[b]	1 mg/kg (not to exceed 80 mg) q8h	IV	2 wk	

HACEK group#

1. Ampicillin	2 g every 4 hr	IV	4 wk	Definitive regimen determined by in vitro susceptibilities.
& gentamicin[b]	1 mg/kg (not to exceed 80 mg) q8h	PO or IV	4 wk	
2. Ceftriaxone[d]	2 g once daily	IV or IM	6 wk	Penicillin allergy.

[a]Dosages are for patients with normal renal function.

[b]Streptomycin 500 mg every 12 hr intramuscularly may be used instead of gentamicin. Gentamicin doses should be adjusted to achieve a peak serum concentration of 3 μg/ml, and streptomycin a peak serum concentration of 20 μg/ml.

[c]Vancomycin peak serum concentrations 1 hour after infusion should be in the range of 30 to 45 μg/ml.

[d]Cephalosporins should be avoided in patients with an immediate type hypersensitivity reaction to penicillin.

[e]This use of rifampin is not listed in the manufacturer's official directive.

[f]*Haemophilus* species, *Actinobacillus actinomycetemcomitans, Cardiobacterium hominis, Eikenella corrodens, Kingella kingii.* MIC = minimum inhibitory concentration.

Therapy of gonococcal infections in hospitalized patients

Disease	Therapy
Acute salpingitis* (pelvic inflammatory disease)	Optimal therapy for acute salpingitis has not been established. Initial therapy should ideally include agents active against gonococci, chlamydiae, genital anaerobes, *Mycoplasma hominis,* and facultative gram-negative rods
Disseminated gonococcal infection	Ceftriaxone, 1 g im or iv every 24 hr daily until improvement occurs, followed by oral cefuroxime axetil, 500 mg twice daily, or amoxicillin, 500 mg with clavulanic acid three times a day, to complete 7 days of therapy
	or
	Ceftizoxime 1 g iv every 8 h daily until improvement occurs, followed by oral cefuroxime axetil, 500 mg twice daily, or amoxicillin, 500 mg with clavulanic acid three times a day, to complete 7 days of therapy
	or
	Ceftizoxime, 1 g iv every 8 hr daily until improvement occurs, followed by oral cefuroxime axetil, 500 mg twice daily, or amoxicillin, 500 mg with clavulanic acid three times a day, to complete 7 days of therapy
	or
	Spectinomycin 2.0 g im twice daily for 3 days (treatment of choice for disseminated infections caused by penicillinase-producing *N. gonorrhoeae,* or PPNG)

*Certain third-generation cephalosporins (e.g., ceftriaxone, cefotaxime, and cefuroxime) and cefoxitin, which are highly active in vitro against PPNG, are currently being evaluated and will probably prove effective for complicated gonococcal infections caused by PPNG, as well as for penicillin-allergic patients with complicated gonococcal infections.

Gonococcal infections, hospitalized patient

Suggested initial drug therapy based on suspected site of origin of gram-negative bacteremia*

Site	Antibiotics	Comment
Urinary tract	—Ampicillin† plus aminoglycoside‡	Combination also covers enterococcus
Respiratory tract:		
Community-acquired	—Erythromycin† and third-generation cephalosporin§ OR first- or second-generation cephalosporin‖ plus aminoglycoside	Gram-negative bacteria cause 10%–20% community pneumonias requiring hospitalization. *Haemophilus influenzae*, *Klebsiella pneumoniae*, and others implicated. Consider *Legionella* if elderly or immunosuppressed.
Hospital-acquired	—Anti-pseudomonal beta-lactam** plus aminoglycoside	Must treat for more resistant organisms including *P. aeruginosa*
Intra-abdominal and biliary tract	—Ticarcillin-clavulanate† plus aminoglycoside OR —Imipenem plus aminoglycoside	Use regimen active against enteric gram-negative bacteria and anaerobes
Burns	—Anti-pseudomonal beta-lactam plus aminoglycoside	Choose agent with greatest anti-peudomonal activity at particular hospital
Catheter infection	—Vancomycin† plus ceftazidime OR —Vancomycin plus aminoglycoside	Include vancomycin for methicillin-resistant staphylococci
Granulocytopenia	—Anti-pseudomonal beta-lactam plus aminoglycoside	Add vancomycin for *Staphylococcus* species if intravascular catheter present

*If source unknown, consider imipenem or ticarcillin-clavulanate plus aminoglycoside. Add vancomycin if gram-positive infection is a consideration.
†Others: Ampicillin 1-2 g every 4-6 hr; erythromycin 0.5-1 g every 6 hr; ticarcillin-clavulanate 3.1 g every 4-8 hr; vancomycin 1 g every 12 hr.
‡Gentamicin, tobramycin 3-5 mg/kg/day divided every 8 hr; amikacin 15 mg/kg/day divided every 8 hr. Must adjust for renal dysfunction.
§Cefotaxime 1-2 g every 6-8 hr; ceftriaxone 1-2 g every 24 hr; ceftazidime 1-2 g every 8 hr.
‖Cefazolin 1 g every 8 hr; cephalothin 1-2 g every 4-6 hr; cefuroxime 1 g every 8 hr.
**Piperacillin, mezlocillin, ticarcillin 3 g every 4 hr; ceftazidime 1-2 g every 8 hr; imipenem 500 mg every 6 hr.

Tailored therapy for advanced heart failure

1. Measurement of baseline hemodynamics
2. Intravenous nitroprusside and diuretics tailored to hemodynamic goals:

PCW $\leq$ 15 mm Hg	RA $\leq$ 8 mm Hg
SVR $\leq$ 1200 dynes-sec-cm^{-5}	SBP $\leq$ 80 mm Hg

3. Definition of optimal hemodynamics by 24-48 hours
4. Titration of high-dose oral vasodilators as nitroprusside weaned
       captopril and isosorbide dinitrate
       occasional addition of hydralazine
5. Monitored ambulation and diuretic adjustment for 24-48 hours
6. Maintenance digoxin levels 1.0-2.0 ng/dl if no contraindication
7. Detailed patient education including sodium restriction
8. Flexible outpatient diuretic regimen including intermittent metolazone
9. Progressive walking program
10. Vigilant follow-up

RA = right atrial pressure, PCW = pulmonary capillary wedge pressure, SBP = systolic blood pressure, SVR = systemic vascular resistance

Chemotherapy of herpesvirus infections

Virus	Host	Disease	Drug
Herpes simplex	Normal or immunocompromised	Initial genital, orofacial, or other mucocutaneous infection	Acyclovir Acyclovir Acyclovir
		Recurrent genital, orofacial, or other	Acyclovir Acyclovir Acyclovir
		Encephalitis	Vidarabine Acyclovir
		Disseminated infection in the neonate	Vidarabine Acyclovir
		Keratitis	Idoxuridine Vidarabine Trifluorothymidine Acyclovir
	Immunocompromised	Resistant to acyclovir	Acyclovir Foscarnet Vidarabine

| Route | Treatment vs. prophylaxis | Approx. response to drug* | | Comments |
		Virus shedding	Clinical response	
Topical	Treatment	++	+	Excellent documentation
IV	Treatment	++++	+++	for genital infection;
Oral	Treatment	+++	+++	poor for other sites of infection. Oral or intravenous therapy should be employed in every case of initial infection
Topical	Treatment	+/0	0	Excellent documentation
Oral	Treatment	++	++	for genital infection;
Oral	Prophylaxis	N/A	+++	fair for recurrences at other sites
IV	Treatment	N/A	++	Acyclovir has been
IV	Treatment	N/A	+++	shown to be superior to vidarabine in two comparative clinical trials
IV	Treatment	+++	+++	Acyclovir and vidarabine
IV	Treatment	+++	+++	are comparable
Topical	Treatment	+++	+++	Activity of these drugs topically is approximately equivalent
Contin-	Treatment	++	+++	Acyclovir-resistant virus
uous	Treatment	+++	+++	often relapses after
infusion	Treatment	+	+	foscarnet therapy
IV				
IV				

Chemotherapy of herpesvirus infections

Virus	Host	Disease	Drug
Varicella zoster	Normal	Chickenpox (initial infection	Acyclovir
		Zoster	Acyclovir
			Acyclovir
	Immunocompro-mised	Chickenpox	Vidarabine
			Acyclovir
		Zoster	Vidarabine
			Interferon
			Acyclovir
			Foscarnet

Route	Treatment vs. prophylaxis	Approx. response to drug*		Comments
		Virus shedding	**Clinical response**	
Oral	Treatment	++	++	Reduces severity when begun within 24 hours
IV	Treatment	+++	+++	No effect on postherpetic neuralgia. High dose resulted in significant toxicity. Most experts recommend no treatment
Oral	Treatment	+++	+++	
IV	Treatment	+++	++	Acyclovir is more effective
IV	Treatment	++++	+++	
IV	Treatment	+++	++	No comparative studies; most authorities prefer
IV/IM	Treatment	+++	++	acyclovir (less toxic;
IV	Treatment	+++	++	possibly more effective)
IV	Treatment	+++	+++	
				Foscarnet used for acyclovir resistant virus

Continued.

Chemotherapy of herpesvirus infections

Virus	Host	Disease	Drug
Epstein-Barr virus	Immunocompromised	Lymphoma or progressive infection	Acyclovir
Cytomegalovirus	Immunocompromised	Various (retinitis, colitis, esophagitis, pneumonitis, etc.)	Acyclovir Ganciclovir Foscarnet

*0, no effect; + + + +, maximum effect.

Herpesvirus infections—cont'd

Route	Treatment vs. prophylaxis	Approx. response to drug*		Comments
		Virus shedding	**Clinical response**	
IV	Treatment	+/0	+/0	Documentation of clinical efficacy is poor
IV/Oral	Prophylaxis	++	++	IV or high dose oral acyclovir reduces rate of CMV disease in transplant recipients
IV	Treatment	++	+++	Ganciclovir treatment reduces rate of pneumonia in marrow recipients with CMV in bronchial lavage; ganciclovir and foscarnet equally effective in controlled trials for retinitis; ganciclovir probably effective for other forms of CMV disease
IV	Treatment	++	+++	

Chemotherapeutic regimens useful in the treatment of Hodgkin's disease

Regimen*	Dose	1	2	3	4	5	6	7	8	9	10	11	12	13	14	15
MOPP																
M = nitrogen mustard	6 mg/m² iv	x							x							
O = vincristine (Oncovin)	1.4 mg/m² iv	x							x							
P = procarbazine	100 mg/m² po	x	x	x	x	x	x	x	x	x	x	x	x	x	x	
P = prednisone	40 mg/m² po	x	x	x	x	x	x	x	x	x	x	x	x	x	x	
ABVD																
A = doxorubicin (Adriamycin)	25 mg/m² iv	x														x
B = bleomycin	10 mg/m² iv	x														x
V = vinblastine	6 mg/m² iv	x														x
D = dacarbazine (DTIC)	375 mg/m² iv	x														x
MOPP/ABVD	Monthly courses alternating two regimens															

Schedule (days)

MOP-BAP

Drug	Dose	1	2	3	4	5	6	7	8	9	10	11	12	13	14
M = nitrogen mustard	6 mg/m² iv	x													
O = vincristine (Oncovin)	1.4 mg/m² iv (max. 2 mg)	x													
P = procarbazine	100 mg/m² po		x	x	x	x	x	x					x		
B = bleomycin	2 mg/m² iv	x							x						
A = doxorubicin (Adriamycin)	30 mg/m² iv								x						
P = prednisone	40 mg/m² po		x	x	x	x	x	x		x	x	x	x		

MOPP-ABV (repeat every 4 weeks)

Drug	Dose	1	2	3	4	5	6	7	8	9	10	11	12	13	14
M = nitrogen mustard	6 mg/m² iv	x													
O = vincristine (Oncovin)	1.4 mg/m² iv (max. 2 mg)	x													
P = procarbazine	100 mg/m² po	x	x	x	x	x	x	x							
P = prednisone	40 mg/m² po	x	x	x	x	x	x	x	x	x	x	x	x	x	x
A = doxorubicin (Adriamycin)	35 mg/m² iv								x						
B = bleomycin	10 mg/m² iv								x						
V = vinblastine	6 mg/m² iv								x						

*MOPP is the standard regimen most often used, and ABVD is the regimen most often used for MOPP failures. MOPP/ABVD is a program that has produced superior results to MOPP alone in one trial. MOP-BAP was shown to be superior to MOPP-bleomycin in one trial. MOPP-ABV is commonly used, but a comparative trial with MOPP has not been completed. In general, each regimen is repeated on a 4 week basis. Most physicians administer a maximum of 2 mg of vincristine per dose in these regimens.

Emergency therapy of hyperkalemia

Therapeutic agent and mechanisms of action	Dose and administration	Onset	Duration
Antagonize cardiac effects			
Calcium gluconate 10%	10-30 ml IV	1 minute	30-60 minutes
Redistribution			
Glucose and insulin	50 g glucose IV hourly	5-10 minutes	2 hours
	5 units regular insulin q15min		
Sodium bicarbonate	50-100 mEq IV	2 hours	3-6 hours
Albuterol	10-20 mg by inhaler	30 minutes	2 hours
Removal			
Sodium polystyrene sulfonate (Kayexalate)	15-60 g with sorbitol orally or 50-100 g with retention enema (hold for 30-60 min)	1-2 hours	
Hemodialysis	Much more effective than peritoneal dialysis	Immediate	
Diuretics ("loop active")		At onset of diuresis	
Furosemide	40-240 mg IV over 30 min		
Ethacrynic acid	50-100 mg IV over 30 min		
Bumetanide	1-8 mg IV over 30 min		

Parenteral drugs for treatment of hypertensive emergency (in order of rapidity of action)

Drug	Dosage	Onset of action	Adverse effects
Vasodilators			
Nitroprusside (Nipride, Nitropress)	0.25-10 μg/kg/min as IV infusion	Instantaneous	Nausea, vomiting, muscle twitching, sweating, thiocyanate intoxication
Nitroglycerin	5-100 μg/min as IV infusion	2-5 min	Tachycardia, flushing, headache, vomiting, methemoglobinemia
Diazoxide (Hyperstat)	50-100 mg/IV bolus repeated, or 15-30 mg/min by IV infusion	2-4 min	Nausea, hypotension, flushing, tachycardia, chest pain
Hydralazine (Apresoline)	10-20 mg IV 10-50 mg IM	10-20 min 20-30 min	Tachycardia, flushing, headache, vomiting, aggravation of angina
Enalapril (Vasotec IV)	1.25-5 mg q 6 hr	15 min	Precipitous fall in BP in high renin states; response variable
Nicardipine	5-10 mg/hr IV	10 min	Tachycardia, headache, flushing, local phlebitis
Adrenergic inhibitors			
Phentolamine (Regitine)	5-15 mg IV	1-2 min	Tachycardia, flushing
Trimethaphan (Arfonad)	0.5-5 mg/min as IV infusion	1-5 min	Paresis of bowel and bladder, orthostatic hypotension, blurred vision, dry mouth
Esmolol (Brevibloc)	500 μg/kg/min for 4 min, then 150-300 μg/kg/min IV	1-2 min	Hypotension
Propranolol (Inderal)	1-10 mg load; 3 ng/hr	1-2 min	Beta blocker side effects, e.g., bronchospasm, decreased cardiac output
Labetalol (Normodyne, Trandate)	20-80 mg IV bolus every 10 min 2 mg/min IV infusion	5-10 min	Vomiting, scalp tingling, burning in throat, postural hypotension. dizziness, nausea

Treatment of hyponatremia

A. **Hypertonic hyponatremia:** Replace salt losses from the osmotic diuresis and treat the underlying disorder (e.g., hyperglycemia, exposure to mannitol, glycine)

B. **Isotonic hyponatremia:** Recognize the potential roles of hyperproteinemia and hyperlipidemia, or exposure to isotonic, sodium-free solutions (e.g., 5% dextrose)

C. **Hypotonic hyponatremia:**
   1. **Hypovolemic states:** Restore ECF volume status with isotonic saline and treat underlying gastrointestinal, adrenal, renal conditions
   2. **Hypervolemic states:** Water restriction and treatment of the underlying disorders (e.g., congestive heart failure, liver disease, nephrosis)
   3. **Isovolemic states:**
      a. **Asymptomatic:**
         Water restriction, increased sodium intake with furosemide, (demeclocycline, lithium, if antagonism of ADH is deemed necessary)
      b. **Symptomatic:**
         (i) Recognize predisposing causes for demyelination: women, elderly, alcoholism, liver disease, malnutrition.
         (ii) 3% saline with furosemide to achieve initial correction rates of 1.0 mEq/L/hr. Continue until symptoms abate or for 4 to 5 hours and then slow the rate of correction so as not to exceed increases of more than 10 to 15 mEq/L/24 hr.

Chemotherapeutic regimens useful in the treatment of malignant lymphomas

Regimen*	Dose	1	2	3	4	5	6	7	8	9	10	11	12	13	14	15
CVP (repeat every 21 days)																
C = cyclophosphamide	400 mg/m² po	x	x	x	x	x										
V = vincristine	1.4 mg/m² iv (max. 2.0 mg)	x														
P = prednisone	100 mg po	x	x	x	x	x										
C-MOPP (repeat every 28 days)																
C = cyclophosphamide	650 mg/m² iv	x							x							
O = vincristine (Oncovin)	1.4 mg/m² iv	x							x							
P = procarbazine	100 mg/m² po	x	x	x	x	x	x	x	x	x	x	x	x	x	x	
P = prednisone	40 mg/m² po	x	x	x	x	x	x	x	x	x	x	x	x	x	x	
CHOP (repeat every 21 days)																
C = cyclophosphamide	750 mg/m² iv	x														
H = doxorubicin (Adriamycin)	50 mg/m² iv	x														
O = vincristine (Oncovin)	1.4 mg/m² iv	x														
P = prednisone	100 mg iv	x	x	x	x	x										

*CVP and single-agent chlorambucil are the standard regimens most often used for favorable histologic subtypes of malignant lymphoma. CHOP is the standard regimen most often used for intermediate grades of unfavorable histologic subtypes. C-MOPP is useful for patients with unfavorable histologic types who have pre-existing heart disease, for whom doxorubicin may be contraindicated. Regimens for the high grades of unfavorable histologic subtypes have not been standardized.

Antibiotics of choice for bacterial meningitis

Organism	Antibiotic(s) of choice	Alternatives
N. meningitidis	Penicillin G	Ampicillin, chloramphenicol, cefuroxime, third-generation cephalosporin
S. pneumoniae	Penicillin G	Same as above, vancomycin
H. influenzae (beta-lactamase—negative)	Ampicillin	Chloramphenicol, cefuroxime, third-generation cephalosporin
H. influenzae (beta-lactamase—positive)	Cefotaxime or ceftriaxone	Chloramphenicol, cefuroxime
Enterobacteriaceae	Third-generation cephalosporin	Aminoglycosides, extended-spectrum penicillins, aztreonam, quinolones
P. aeruginosa	Ceftazidime (? plus an aminoglycoside*)	Extended-spectrum penicillin plus an aminoglycoside, aztreonam, quinolones
S. agalactiae	Penicillin G or ampicillin (? plus an aminoglycoside*)	Third-generation cephalosporin, chloramphenicol
L. monocytogenes	Ampicillin (? plus an aminoglycoside*)	Trimethoprim-sulfamethoxazole, chloramphenicol
S. aureus (methicillin-sensitive)	Nafcillin or oxacillin	Vancomycin (? plus rifampin)
S. aureus (methicillin-resistant)	Vancomycin	Trimethoprim-sulfamethoxazole, quinolones (?)
S. epidermidis	Vancomycin (? plus rifampin)	Penicillin G
M. tuberculosis	Isoniazid plus rifampin (? plus ethambutol or pyrazinamide)	
Candida sp.	Amphotericin B	Fluconazole
C. neoformans	Amphotericin B (? plus 5-fluorocytosine)	Fluconazole
C. immitis	Amphotericin B†	Fluconazole

*Value of aminoglycoside addition unproved.
†Intraventricular administration is usually required in addition to systemic route.

Empiric therapy of purulent meningitis

Age	Standard therapies	Alternative therapies
0-3 wk	Ampicillin plus cefotaxime	Ampicillin plus an aminoglycoside
4-12 wk	Cefotaxime or ceftriaxone plus ampicillin	
3 mo-18 yr	Cefotaxime or ceftriaxone	Cefuroxime, ampicillin, chloramphenicol, ampicillin plus chloramphenicol
18 yr-50 yr	Cefotaxime or ceftriaxone	Chloramphenicol
>50 yr	Third-generation cephalosporin plus ampicillin	Ampicillin plus an aminoglycoside, trimethoprim-sulfamethoxazole

Drugs used in the treatment of mycobacterial disease

Antituberculosis drugs	Adult dosage		Most common side effects	Tests for side effects
	Daily	Twice weekly		
Primary				
Isoniazid	5-10 mg/kg, up to 300 mg P.O. or I.M.	15 mg/kg P.O. or I.M.	Peripheral neuritis, hepatitis, hypersensitivity	AST-ALT
Ethambutol	15-25 mg/kg P.O.	50 mg/kg P.O.	Optic neuritis (reversible with discontinuation of drugs: very rare at 15 mg/kg), skin rash	Red-green color discrimination and visual acuity*
Rifampin	10-15 mg/kg, up to 600 mg P.O.	600 mg P.O.	Hepatitis, febrile reaction, purpura (rare), drug interactions	AST-ALT
Streptomycin	15 mg/kg, up to 1 g I.M.	15-25 mg/kg I.M.	VIIIth nerve damage (vestibular), nephrotoxicity	Vestibular function, audiograms,* BUN, and creatinine
Pyrazinamide	25 mg/kg, up to 2 g P.O.		Hyperuricemia, hepatotoxicity	Uric acid, AST-ALT

Secondary			
Capreomycin	12-15 mg/kg, up to 1 g I.M.	VIIIth nerve damage (auditory), nephrotoxicity, vestibular toxicity (rare)	Vestibular function, audiograms,* BUN, and creatinine
Kanamycin	12-15 mg/kg, up to 1 g I.M.	VIIIth nerve damage (auditory), nephrotoxicity, vestibular toxicity (rare)	Vestibular function, audiograms,* BUN, and creatinine
Amikacin	15 mg/kg	Auditory, vestibulary, renal	Same as other aminoglycosides
Ethionamide	15 mg/kg, up to 1 g P.O.	GI disturbance, hepatotoxicity, hypersensitivity	AST-ALT
p-Aminosalicylic acid (aminosalicylic acid)	150 mg/kg, up to 12 g P.O.	GI disturbance, hypersensitivity, hepatotoxicity, sodium load	AST-ALT
Cycloserine	15 mg/kg, up to 1 g P.O.	Psychosis, personality changes, convulsions, rash	
Ofloxacin	600 mg	Rash, GI	
Ciprofloxacin	500-700 mg	GI, CNS	

BUN, blood urea nitrogen; AST, serum aspartate aminotransferase; ALT, serum alanine aminotransferase.

*Determine at the start of treatment.

Treatment of myxedema coma

Thyroid hormone administration
   l-thyroxine 300 to 500 μ IV then 100 μ daily
or
   Triiodothyronine 25 to 50 μ IV then 25 μ q 8 h
Intravenous fluids
Gentle warming
Glucocorticoid 50-100 mg hydrocortisone q 8 h
Antibiotics for suspected infection
Respiratory support

Drug regimens for treatment of patients with *P. carinii* infections				
Regimen	Adult total daily dosage	Route	Interval	Dose-limiting side effects
Recommended regimens				
Trimethoprim (TMP)/ sulfamethoxazole (SMX)	15-20 mg/kg (TMP) 75-100 mg/kg (SMX)	PO or IV	q6-8h	Rash, nausea, neutropenia, anemia, hepatitis, azotemia, decreased platelet count
Pentamidine isethionate	3-4 mg/kg	IV or IM	q24h	Azotemia, neutropenia, hypoglycemia, hepatitis, orthostasis, diabetes mellitus
Atovaquone*	2250mg	PO	q8h	Rash, hepatitis, neutropenia, nausea
Regimens under study				
Dapsone plus TMP	100 mg 12-15 mg/kg	PO PO	q24h q6-8h	Rash, nausea, methemoglobinemia, anemia, hepatitis, neutropenia
Clindamycin plus primaquine	1800 mg 30 mg (base)	PO or IV PO	q8h q24h	Rash, diarrhea, neutropenia, nausea
Pentamidine isethionate	600 mg	Aerosolized	q24h	Bronchospasm
Trimetrexate plus folinic acid	45 mg/m² 80 mg/m²	IV PO or IV	q24h q24h	Neutropenia, decreased platelet count, anemia, hepatitis

PO, Oral; IV, intravenous; IM, intramuscular; q, every; h, hours.
*Indicated for treatment of TMP/SMX–intolerant patients.

Pneumocystis carinii infections

Treatment of community-acquired pneumonia

Cause	Primary antibiotic	Alternative antibiotic
S. pneumoniae	Hospitalized cefuroxime 750 mg q12h penicillin V, 500 mg qid po until afebrile for 4 d	Erythromycin, 500 mg po or IV q6h, or cefotaxime or ceftriaxone
Aerobic gram-negative bacilli		
H. influenzae	Cefuroxime or a third-generation cephalosporin for 10-14 days (switch to ampicillin if sensitve)	Trimethoprim-sulfamethoxazole (see below) Fluoroquinolone
S. aureus	Nafcillin or oxacillin, 2 g IV q1 to 6h for 14 days	Vancomycin, 1 g IV q12h
S. pyogenes	Aqueous procaine penicillin G, 600,000 U IM q12h until afebrile for 3 days then penicillin V, 500 mg po qid for 2-3 wk	Erythromycin 500 mg po or IV q6h, or a cephalosporin
Necrotizing pneumonia or lung abscess	Clindamycin, 600 mg IV q8h until afebrile, then 300 mg po q8h; penicillin G, 10-20 million U/d IV until response, then penicillin V, 500-750 mg qid for 6-12 wk	Cefoxitin, 2 g IV q6h
M. pneumoniae	Erythromycin, 250-500 mg po q6h for 10-14 days, clarithromycin, 500 mg po q12h, or azithromycin, 250 mg po qd for 10 d	Tetracycline, 250-500 mg po q6h
L. pneumophila	Erythromycin, 1 g IV q6h until afebrile for 48 h, then 500 mg po q6h for total 3 wk or Rifampin 600 mg po qd for severely ill	Ciprofloxacin, 750 mg po q12h or Ofloxacin, 400 mg po q12h
P. carinii	Trimethoprim-sulfamethoxazole, 20 mg trimethoprim/100 mg sulfamethoxazole/kg/d IV in four divided doses daily, or pentamidine 4 mg/kg/day IV	Trimethoprim plus dapsone

Specific antidotes

Antidote	Poison	Dosages
Naloxone	Opiates (heroin, meperidine, propoxyphene, pentazocine, diphenoxylate)	Loading dose: From 0.4 to 2.0 mg iv; repeat in 2-5 min as necessary Maintenance dose: sufficient to maintain desired level of consciousness
Atropine	Organophosphates	Loading dose: 2 mg iv or im every 2-5 min until hypersalivation is controlled Maintenance dose: sufficient to suppress hypersalivation
Pralidoxime	Organophosphates	Loading dose: 1-2 g iv Maintenance dose: 1-2 g after 2-3 hr
Ethanol	Methanol, ethylene glycol	Loading dose: 0.6-0.7 g/kg Maintenance dose: sufficient EtOH* to maintain serum alcohol level at 100 mg/dl (approximately 125 mg/kg/hr) until methanol, ethylene glycol concentration < 10 mg/dl
Amyl nitrite Sodium nitrite Sodium thiosulfate	Cyanide	Amyl nitrite ampuls inhaled every 2-3 min; monitor blood pressure; then 10 ml 3% sodium nitrite iv over 5 min; then 50 ml 25% sodium thiosulfate over 10 min
Deferoxamine	Iron salts	Hypotensive patients: 10 mg/kg/hr iv for 4 hr; then 5 mg/kg/hr iv for 8 hr, then 2-5 mg/kg/hr iv until serum iron level is less than 100 μ/dl Normotensive patients: 40 mg/kg im every 4-12 hr (total dose should not exceed 6 g/24 hr)
N-Acetylcysteine	Acetaminophen	140 mg/kg po then 70 mg/kg every 4 hr po for 17 doses
Oxygen	Carbon monoxide	100% by face mask or hyperbaric
Flumazenil	Benzodiazepines	Loading dose: 1-5 mg iv Maintenance dose: sufficient to maintain desired level of consciousness

*EtOH, ethylalcohol or ethanol.

Antibiotic therapy of acute septic arthritis in adults*

Organism	Duration (days)	Drug of choice	Alternative drug/dose
Streptococci (nonenterococcal) or pneumococci	14	Penicillin G, 150,000 units/kg/d I.V. in q4h doses	Cephalothin,† 150 mg/kg/d I.V. in q4h doses
Enterococci	28	Penicillin G, 150,000 units/kg/d I.V. in q4h doses, *plus* gentamicin,‡ 3–5 mg/kg/d I.M. or I.V. in q8h doses	Vancomycin, 30 mg/kg/d I.V. in q6h doses, *plus* gentamicin,‡ in doses noted
Staphylococcus aureus	28–42	Nafcillin or oxacillin, 150 mg/kg/d I.V. in q4h doses	Vancomycin or cephalothin† in doses noted above
S. aureus or Staphylococcus epidermidis (methicillin-resistant)	28–42	Vancomycin, 30 mg/kg/d I.V. in q6h doses	—
Pseudomonas aeruginosa	42	Tobramycin,‡ 5–6 mg/kg/d I.M. or I.V. in q8h doses, *plus* ticarcillin, 250–300 mg/kg/d I.V. in q4h doses	An aminoglycoside‡ *plus* piperacillin, mezlocillin, or ceftazidine in full doses may be used if resistance encountered
Other facultative gram-negative bacilli (susceptibility permitting)	28–42	Gentamicin,‡ 5–6 mg/kg/d I.M. or I.V. in q8h doses, *plus* a broad-spectrum penicillin (mezlocillin or piperacillin) or a third-generation cephalosporin (cefotaxime, ceftizoxime, or ceftazidine) in doses for life-threatening infection	Tobramycin,‡ netilmicin,‡ or amikacin,‡ *plus* either a third-generation cephalosporin, piperacillin, or mezlocillin, each in doses for life-threatening infection

*Recommended doses assume normal renal function. Many agents require dose adjustments if renal function is reduced.
†An equivalent cephalosporin antibiotic and dose may be used.
‡Lean body weight used to calculate doses.

Management of shock

I. Initial resuscitation and supportive measures
    A. Establish effective ventilation and adequate oxygenation (O_2 tension >70 mm Hg).
    B. Restore viable central pulses with dopamine or norepinephrine.
    C. If hypovolemia is suspected, begin rapid volume replacement.
    D. Treat pain, arrhythmias, and acid-base abnormalities.
II. Pharmacologic therapy
    A. Initiate volume replacement to optimize cardiac filling pressures and cardiac output.
    B. Administer vasoactive-inotropic drugs (dopamine, norepinephrine) to maintain mean arterial pressure at 65 to 70 mm Hg and improve cardiac output.
    C. Administer vasodilator drugs (nitroprusside, phentolamine) to improve tissue perfusion in the patient with excessive vasoconstriction. Do not use these drugs unless hypovolemia is corrected and systolic blood pressure is ≥80 mm Hg.
    D. Administer diuretics (furosemide, ethacrynic acid) to reduce elevated cardiac filling pressures, reduce pulmonary edema, and increase urine flow.
III. Mechanical circulatory assist (cardiogenic shock): use in conjunction with pharmacologic therapy to improve coronary perfusion and cardiac performance.
IV. Definitive therapy: establish underlying cause(s) and institute specific therapy.

Management of generalized status epilepticus in adults

1. Observe seizures briefly while getting history: consider pseudoseizures.
2. Give diazepam, 10 mg I.V., to arrest convulsion.
3. Start I.V.s; intubate trachea; draw blood samples; give glucose 25 g, thiamine 50 mg, calcium gluconate 100 mg I.V.
Reexamine briefly.
4. Begin phenytoin infusion, 18 mg/kg, 50 mg/min maximum rate, with ECG and BP monitoring: expect convulsions to subside during or soon after phenytoin loading.
5. If seizures are uncontrolled, give phenobarbital 3-5 mg/kg I.V. over 5–10 min; expect prompt control.
6. If seizures are uncontrolled, assess plasma AED levels (phenytoin >30, phenobarbital >45), plasma glucose, oxygenation, and acidosis; give bicarbonate; get experienced neurologic advice.
7. If seizures are controlled, give maintenance AED.

Treatment of syphilis

Diagnosis	Recommended treatment	Alternative penicillin treatment	In penicillin allergy
Sexual contact to infectious syphilis (primary, secondary, early latent)	Benzathine penicillin G, 2.4 million U I.M. at a single treatment session	Procaine penicillin G, 600,000 U I.M. daily for 8 days	Tetracycline hydrochloride, 500 mg orally 4 times daily for 15 days or Doxycycline, 200 mg orally twice daily for 15 days or Ceftriaxone, 250 mg I.M. once*†
Early syphilis (primary, secondary, or latent of less than 1 year duration)	Benzathine penicillin G, 2.4 million U I.M. at a single treatment session	Procaine penicillin G, 600,000 U I.M. daily for 8 days	Tetracycline hydrochloride, 500 mg orally 4 times daily for 15 days or Doxycycline, 200 mg orally twice daily for 15 days or Ceftriaxone, 250 mg I.M. once daily for 10 days*

Condition			
Syphilis of more than 1 year duration including latent, late benign, and cardiovascular	Benzathine penicillin G, 2.4 million U I.M. at weekly intervals for three doses	Procaine penicillin G, 600,000 U I.M. daily for 15 days	Doxycycline, 200 mg orally twice daily for 21 days or Ceftriaxone, 250 mg I.M. once daily for 14 days*
Neurosyphilis (asymptomatic paresis, tabes)	Aqueous crystalline penicillin G, 20 million U daily I.V. by continuous infusion or in divided doses, q4h for 15 d‡	Procaine penicillin G, 600,000 U I.M. daily for 15 days	Doxycycline, 200 mg orally twice daily for 21 days or Ceftriaxone, 1 g I.V. once daily for 14 days*
Pregnancy	Regimen appropriate for stage of maternal syphilis	Regimen appropriate for stage of maternal syphilis	Ceftriaxone*·§ or Erythromycin† regimen appropriate for stage of maternal syphilis

*Ceftriaxone should not be used if there is a history of anaphylaxis to penicillin.

†This regimen appears to abort most but not all cases of incubating syphilis.

‡Some experts have suggested following this regimen with benzathine penicillin G as administered for syphilis of more than one year's duration.

§The treatment of syphilis in the penicillin-allergic pregnant patient is very difficult, and desensitization may be required. Consultation with an expert is recommended.

Thrombolytic therapy for patients with MI

Indications

Ongoing Q wave MI longer than 30 minutes and less than 6 hours manifested by S-T segment elevation of 1 mV or greater in two or more ECG leads

Ongoing Q wave MI longer than 6 and less than 24 hours with continued ischemic pain

Chest pain and S-T depression in anterior precordial leads coupled with imaging test demonstrating posterior left ventricular wall motion abnormality

Patient consent

Absence of absolute contraindications

Contraindications

Absolute

    Active bleeding

    Recent ($<$ 6 weeks) major surgical procedure or arterial puncture in noncompressible area or recent major trauma

    Symptomatic cerebrovascular disease or intracranial pathologic condition

Relative

    History of gastrointestinal bleeding or active ulcer disease

    Recent (6 months) administration of streptokinase or allergy to this drug (applies only to streptokinase)

    Cardiogenic shock

    History of bleeding diathesis

    Remote history of cerebrovascular disease

    Prolonged cardiopulmonary resuscitation

Treatment of thyroid storm

Propranolol—160 mg/day orally in 4 divided doses; or 1 mg *slowly* IV q 4 h under careful monitoring

IV glucose solutions

Correction of dehydration and electrolyte imbalance

Iodide-30 drops Lugol's solution daily orally in 3 or 4 divided doses; or 1 to 2 g sodium iodine slowly by IV drip

Propylthiouracil—900 to 1200 mg/day orally or by gastric tube

Cooling blanket for hyperthermia

Plasmapheresis to lower T_4 and T_3 levels (in selected cases)

Digitalis if necessary

Treatment of underlying disease (e.g., infection)

Corticosteroid—100 mg hydrocortisone IV q 8 hr

Definitive therapy after control of the crisis—ablation of the thyroid gland with ^{131}I or surgery.

Medication Comparison Tables

Antiepileptic drugs in common use

Generic name	Trade name	Typical adult dose range (mg/day)	Target plasma level (µg/ml)	Serum half-life (h)	Side effects	
					Dose-dependent	Idiosyncratic
Carbamazepine	Tegretol	600-1200	4-12	15	Ataxia, diplopia, nystagmus	Hyponatremia, rash, aplastic anemia
Phenytoin	Dilantin	300-400	10-20	24	Ataxia, nystagmus, gingival hyperplasia	Rash, lymphadenopathy
Valproate	Depakote	1000-2500	50-100	12	Gastric distress, alopecia, weight gain	Tremor, hepatic failure, decreased platelets
Phenobarbital	Luminal	60-180	15-30	96	Sedation, ataxia, blurred vision	Hyperactivity
Primidone	Mysoline	500-1500	5-10	16	Sedation, ataxia, blurred vision	
Ethosuximide	Zarontin	750-1500	40-100	36	Ataxia, sedation, gastric distress, headache	Rash
Clonazepam	Klonopin	15-20	.01-.05	30	Sedation, ataxia	

Antidepressant drugs

Drug	Typical full dose	Dosage range	Notes
Tertiary amine tricyclic:			
Amitriptyline	100-200	10-300	1 2 3 4
Doxepin	100-200	10-300	1 2 3 4
Imipramine	100-200	10-300	1 2 3 4
Trimipramine	100-200	25-300	1 2 3 4
Clomipramine	100-200	25-250	1 2 3 4
Secondary amine tricyclic:			
Desipramine	100-200	10-300	3 4
Nortriptyline	50-100	10-150	4
Protriptyline	20-30	10-60	1 4 5
Amoxapine	100-200	25-300	3 4 5 6
Maprotiline	100-200	25-225	2 3 4 7
Trazodone	200-400	50-600	2 3
Bupropion	300-400	150-450	5 7
Serotonin reuptake inhibitors:			
Fluoxetine	20-60	5-80	5
Sertraline	50-150	25-200	8
Paroxetine	20-60	10-60	
MAO inhibitors:			
Phenelzine	45-60	30-90	3 5 9
Tranylcypromine	30-40	20-60	3 5 9

NOTES
1. Relatively high anticholinergic effects
2. Relatively high sedation
3. Relatively high rate of orthostatic hypotension
4. Quinidine-like effects on cardiac conduction
5. Prominent stimulating effect; may cause agitation early in treatment
6. Neuroleptic effects—risk of tardive dyskinesia and parkinsonism
7. Relatively high seizure risk: raise dosage slowly and avoid single doses >150 mg for bupropion
8. Frequent GI side effects
9. Special diet and drug interaction precautions needed

Comparison of azole antifungal drugs now available

	Ketoconazole	Fluconazole	Itraconazole
Route administered	Oral	Oral/I.V.	Oral only
Achlorhydric effect	Marked	Minimal	Significant
Half-life	5-9 hrs	24-30 hrs	30-42 hrs
Clearance	Hepatic	Renal, largely unchanged	Hepatic, with active metabolite
Usual highest dose*	400 mg/D	400 mg/D	400 mg/D
Drug interactions:			
Phenytoin	+++	++	+++
Rifampin	+++	++	+++
H$_2$ blockers	+++	+	+++
Cyclosporine A	+++	+	++

Differences in spectrum (estimate of overall efficacy, based on noncomparative studies)

Histoplasma	++	++	+++
Coccidioides	+	++	+++
Blastomyces	+++	++	+++
Paracoccidioides	++	++	+++
Sporothrix	+	++	+++
Aspergillus	0	0	+++
Chromomycosis	Unk	Unk	+++
Dematiaceous	Unk	Unk	++
Candida			
Mucosal	++	+++	+++
Dissem.	+	++	Unk
"Meningitis"	+	+++	+++
Toxicity:			
Nausea/vomit	+++	+	+
Hepatic	++	+	+
Endocrine	+++	0	0†

* = All three drugs have been used at more than 1 gram/D, with ketoconazole showing marked gastrointestinal and endocrine effects above 400 per day, and fluconazole showing no clear toxic effects at up to 2 grams per day. Loading doses of 600-800 mg per day can be used for 2-3 days to accelerate achieving steady state.

† = Infrequently seen side effects include edema, hypertension, and hypokalemia, which may be endocrine in cause, although unpublished investigations have not identified an endocrine cause (Graybill JR et al).

Effective oral antihypertensive drugs

Drug	Trade name	Dose range mg/day (frequency)	Side effects
Diuretics (partial list)			
Hydrochlorothiazide	Hydrodiuril Esidrix	12.5-50(1)	Biochemical abnormalities: ↓ potassium, ↑ cholesterol, ↑ glucose Rare: blood dyscrasias, photosensitivity, pancreatitis
Chlorthalidone	Hygroton	12.5-50	
Metolazone	Mykrox, Diulo	0.5-10	
Indapamide	Lozol	2.5	Less if any hypercholesterolemia
Furosemide	Lasix	40-240	Short duration of action
Potassium-sparing agents (plus thiazide)			
Spironolactone	Aldactazide	25-100	Hyperkalemia, gynecomastia
Triamterene	Dyazide, Maxzide	25-100	Hyperkalemia
Amiloride	Moduretic	5-10	Hyperkalemia
Adrenergic inhibitors			
Peripherals:			
Reserpine	Serpasil	0.05-0.25(1)	Sedation, depression
Guanethidine	Ismelin	10-150	Orthostatic hypotension, diarrhea
Guanadrel	Hylorel	10-75	

Central alpha agonists:			
Methyldopa	Aldomet	500-3000(2)	Hepatic and "autoimmune" disorders
Clonidine	Catapres	0.2-1.2(2)	Sedation, dry mouth, "withdrawal"
Guanabenz	Wytensin	8-32(2)	Sedation, dry mouth, "withdrawal"
Guanfacine	Tenex	1-3(1)	Sedation, dry mouth, "withdrawal"
Alpha blockers:			
Doxazosin	Cardura	1-20(1)	Postural hypotension (mainly with first dose), lassitude
Prazosin	Minipress	2-20(2)	
Terazosin	Hytrin	1-20(1)	
Beta blockers:			
Acebutolol	Sectral	200-800(1)	Serious: bronchospasm, congestive heart failure, masking of insulin-induced hypoglycemia, depression
Atenolol	Tenormin	25-100(1-2)	
Betaxolol	Kerlone	5-20(1)	
Carteolol	Cartrol	2.5-10(1)	Less serious: poor peripheral circulation, insomnia, fatigue, decreased exercise tolerance, hypertriglyceridemia, decreased HDL (except with ISA agents)
Metoprolol	Lopressor	50-300(1-2)	
Nadolol	Corgard	40-320(1)	
Penbutolol	Levatol	10-20(1)	
Pindolol	Visken	10-60(2)	
Propranolol	Inderal	40-480(2)	
Timolol	Blocadren	20-60(2)	
Combined alpha and beta blocker:			
Labetalol	Normodyne Trandate	200-1200(2)	Postural hypotension, beta-blocking side effects
Direct vasodilators:			
Hydralazine	Apresoline	50-400(2)	Headaches, tachycardia, lupus syndrome
Minoxidil	Loniten	5-100(1)	Headaches, fluid retention, hirsutism

Effective oral antihypertensive drugs—cont'd

Drug	Trade name	Dose range mg/day (frequency)	Side effects
Calcium entry blockers			
Verapamil (SR)	Isoptin, Calan Verelan	90-480(1-2)	Constipation, conduction defects
Diltiazem (SR and CD)	Cardizem	120-240(1-2)	Nausea, headache, conduction defects
Dihydropyridines:			
Amlodipine	Norvase	2.5-10(1)	Flush, headache, local ankle edema
Felodipine	Plendil	5-20(1)	Flush, headache, local ankle edema
Isradipine	DynaCirc	5-20(2)	Flush, headache, local ankle edema
Nicardipine	Cardene	60-90(2-3)	Flush, headache, local ankle edema
Nifedipine (XL)	Procardia	20-120(1)	Flush, headache, local ankle edema
Converting-enzyme inhibitors			
Benazepril	Lotensin	5-40(1)	Cough, rash, loss of taste
Captopril	Capoten	25-150(2)	Rare: leucopenia, proteinuria
Enalapril	Vasotec	5-40(1-2)	Rare: leucopenia, proteinuria
Fosinopril	Monopril	10-40(1)	Rare: leucopenia, proteinuria
Lisinopril	Prinivil, Zestril	5-40(1)	Rare: leucopenia, proteinuria
Quinapril	Accupril	2.5-10(1)	Rare: leucopenia, proteinuria
Ramipril	Altace	1.25-20(1)	Rare: leucopenia, proteinuria

Dosage of antimicrobial agents

Drug	Normal unit dose (route)	Normal dose interval (h)	Adjusted maximum dose in renal failure			Removal by dialysis
			GFR >50 ml/min	GFR 10-50 ml/min	GFR <10 ml/min	
Aminoglycosides						
Gentamicin, tobramycin*	1.0-1.7 mg/kg (IM,IV)	8	1.0-1.7 mg/kg q(8 × creatinine)h or (1.0-1.7 mg/kg ÷ creatinine) q8h†			Yes(H,P)†
Netilmicin*	1.3-2.2 mg/kg (IM,IV)	8	1.3-2.2 mg/kg q(8 × creatinine)h or (1.3-2.2 mg/kg ÷ creatinine) q8h†			Yes(H,P)§
Kanamycin, amikacin*	5 mg/kg (IM,IV)	8	5 mg/kg q(8 × creatinine)h or (5 mg/kg ÷ creatinine) q8h†			Yes(H,P)‖
Azithromycin	250-500 mg (PO)	24	Unknown	Unknown	Unknown	Unknown
Carbapenems						
Imipenem	0.5-1(IV)	6	0.5 q6h**	0.5 q8-12h	0.25-0.5 q12h††	Yes(H)

Continued.

Dosage of antimicrobial agents—cont'd

Drug	Normal unit dose (route)	Normal dose interval (h)	Adjusted maximum dose in renal failure			Removal by dialysis
			GFR >50 ml/min	GFR 10-50 ml/min	GFR <10 ml/min	
Cephalosporins						
Cefaclor	0.25-0.5 g (PO)	8	NC	NC	NC	Yes(H)
Cefadroxil	0.5-1.0 g (PO)	12	NC	0.5 g q12-24h	0.5 g q36h	Yes(H)
Cefamandole	1-2 g (IM,IV)	4	1-2 g q6h	1-2 g q6-8h	0.5-1.0 g q8-12h	Yes(H), No(P)
Cefazolin	0.5-1.5 g (IM,IV)	8	0.5-1.0 g q8h	0.5-1.0 g q12h	0.5-1.0 g q24-48h	Yes(H), No(P)
Cefixime	400 mg (PO)	24	NC§§	300 mg q24h‖	200 mg q24h***	No(H,P)
Cefmetazole	2 g (IV)	6-12	1-2 g q12h	1-2 g q16-24h	1-2 g q48h	Yes(H)
Cefonicid	1-2 g (IM,IV)	24	NC	1 g q24-48h	0.25-1.0 g q72-120h	No(H)
Cefoperazone	1-3 g (IM,IV)	8	NC	NC	NC	Yes(H)
Cefóranide	0.5-1.0 g (IM,IV)	12	NC	1 g q24-48h	1 g q48-72h	Yes(H)
Cefotaxime	1-2 g (IM,IV)	6	NC	1-2 g q6-12h	1-2 g q12-24h	Yes(H), No(P)
Cefotetan	2 g (IV,IM)	12	NC	1-2 g q12-24h	1-2 g q48h	Yes (H)
Cefoxitin	1-2 g (IM,IV)	4	1-2 g q6h	1-2 g q8-24h	0.5-1.0 g q12-48h	Yes(H), No(P)
Cefprozil	250-500 mg (PO)	12-24	NC	125-250 mg q12-24h‡‡	125-250 mg q12-24h	Yes(H)
Ceftazidime	0.5-2.0 g (IM,IV)	8	0.5-2.0 g q8h	0.5-2.0 g q12-24h	0.5-2.0 g q36-48h	Yes(H,P)
Ceftizoxime	1-2 g (IM,IV)	6	1-2 g q8h	1 q12h	0.5 g q12-24h	Yes(H), No(P)
Ceftriaxone	1-2 g (IM,IV)	12-24	NC	NC	NC	No(H)
Cefuroxime	0.75-1.5 g (IM,IV)	6	NC	0.75-1.5 g q8-12h	0.75 g q24h	Yes(H,P)
Cephalexin	0.25-0.5 g (PO)	6	NC	NC	NC	Yes(H,P)
Cephalothin	1-2 g (IV)	4	1-2 g q6h	1-2 g q6h	1 g q8-12h	Yes(H,P)
Cephapirin	1-2 g (IV)	4	1-2 g q6h	1-2 g q6h	1 g q8-12h	Yes(H,P)

Drug	Dose (Route)	(hr)				Dialysis
Cephradine	1-2 g (IV); 0.25-0.5 g (PO)	4	1-2 g q6h	1 g q6h	1 g q12h	Yes(H,P)
Chloramphenicol	0.25-1.0 g (PO,IV)	6	NC	NC	NC	Yes(H), Not(P)
Clarithromycin	250-500 mg (PO)	12	Unknown	Unknown	Unknown	Unknown
Clindamycin	0.6 g (IM,IV); 0.15-0.3 g (PO)	6-8	NC	NC	NC	No(H,P)
Erythromycin	0.5-1.0 g (IV); 0.25-0.5 g (PO)	6	NC	NC	NC	No(H,P)
Metronidazole	15 mg/kg load (IV), then 7.5 mg/kg (IV)	6	NC	NC	NC	Yes(H), Not(P)
Monobactams						
Aztreonam	1-2 g (IV)	8	NC	1 g q8h	0.5 g q6-12h	Yes(H,P)
Nitrofurantoin	50-100 mg (PO)	6	NC	Avoid	Avoid	Yes(H)
Penicillins						
Amoxicillin	0.25-0.5 g (PO)	8	NC	0.25-0.5 g q12h	0.25 g q12h	Yes(H), No(P)
Ampicillin	0.5-2.0 g (IM,IV)	4	NC	0.5-2.0 g q8h	0.5-2.0 g q12h	Yes(H), No(P)
Ampicillin	0.25-0.5 g (PO)	6	NC	0.25-0.5 g q8h	0.25-0.5 g q12h	
Azlocillin	2-3 g (IM,IV)	4	NC	3 g q6h	3 g q12h	Yes(H), No(P)
Carbenicillin	2-5 g (IM,IV)	4	NC	2-5 g q6h	2 g q8-12h	Yes(H,P)
Indanyl-carbenicillin	0.5-1.0 g (PO)	6	NC	NC	Avoid	
Cloxacillin	0.5-1.0 g (PO)	6	NC	NC	NC	No(H,P)
Dicloxacillin	0.25-0.5 g (PO)	6	NC	NC	NC	No(H,P)
Methicillin	1-2 g (IM,IV)	4	NC	NC	1-2 g q8-12h	No(H,P)
Mezlocillin	2-3 g (IM,IV)	4	NC	3 g q6-8h	2 g q6-8h	Yes(H), No(P)
Nafcillin	1-2 g (IM,IV)	4	NC	NC	NC	No(H,P)
Oxacillin	0.5-1.0 g (PO)	6	NC	NC	NC	No(H,P)

Dosage of antimicrobial agents—cont'd

Drug	Normal unit dose (route)	Normal dose interval (h)	Adjusted maximum dose in renal failure			Removal by dialysis
			GFR >50 ml/min	GFR 10-50 ml/min	GFR <10 ml/min	
Penicillin G	0.4-4.0 million units (IM,IV)	4	NC	NC	2 million units q4h	Yes(H), No(P)
Penicillin V	0.25-0.5 g (PO)	6	NC	NC	NC	Yes(H), No(P)
Piperacillin	2-3 g (IM,IV)	4	NC	3 g q6h	3 g q8h	Yes(H)
Ticarcillin	2-3 g (IM,IV)	4	NC	2-3 g q6h	2 g q12h	Yes(H,P)
Polymyxins						
Polymyxin B	1.5-2.5 mg/kg/day (IV)	Continuous infusion	Avoid	Avoid	Avoid	No(H), Yes(P)
Colistin	0.8-1.7 mg/kg (IM)	8	Avoid	Avoid	Avoid	No(H), Yes(P)
Quinolones						
Nalidixic acid	0.5-1.0 g (PO)	6	NC	NC	Avoid	Unknown
Ciprofloxacin	250-750 mg (PO)	12	NC	250-500 mg q12h†††	250-500 mg q18h‡‡‡	No(<14%) (H,P)
	200-400 mg (IV)	12	NC	200-400 mg q18-24h‡‡‡	200-400 mg q18-24h‡‡‡	No(<14%) (H,P)
Lomefloxacin	400 mg (PO)	24	NC	200 q24h	Unknown	No(<14%) (H,P)
Norfloxacin	400 mg (PO)	12	NC	400 q24h	400 q24h	No(<14%) (H,P)
Ofloxacin	200-400 mg (PO,IV)	12	NC	200-400 mg q24h	100-200 mg q24h	No(<14%) (H,P)

Sulfisoxazole	1 g (PO)	6	NC	1 g q8-12h	1 g q12-24h	Yes(H,P)
Tetracyclines						
Tetracycline	0.25-0.5 g (PO,IV)	6	0.25-0.5 g q8-12h	Avoid	Avoid	No(H,P)
Doxycycline	100 mg (PO,IV)	12-24	NC	NC	NC	No(H,P)
Trimethoprim-sulfamethoxazole	2-3 mg TMP/kg (IV)	6	NC	2-3 mg TMP/kg q12h	Avoid	Yes(H), No(P)
	160/800 mg (PO)	12	NC	160/800 mg q24h	Avoid	
Trimethoprim	100 mg (PO)	12	NC	100 mg q24h	Avoid	Yes(H), No(P)
Vancomycin*	1 g (IV)	12	1 g q24-72h	1 g q72-240h	1 g q240h	No(H,P)

GFR, glomerular filtration rate; H, hemodialysis; P, peritoneal dialysis; NC, no change; TMP, trimethoprim.

*Serum level monitoring is recommended for therapy of the patient with renal impairment.

†When using the latter formula, a normal unit dose is necessary initially.

‡Following an initial loading dose, therapeutic levels can be maintained by administering a dose of 1 mg/kg after each hemodialysis or by adding 5 µg/ml to the peritoneal dialysis fluid.

§Following an initial loading dose, therapeutic levels can be maintained by administering a dose of 1.5 mg/kg after each hemodialysis or by adding 7.5 µg/ml to the peritoneal dialysis fluid.

‖Following an initial loading dose, therapeutic levels can be maintained by administering a dose of 3.5 mg/kg after each hemodialysis or by adding 20 µg/ml to the peritoneal dialysis fluid.

**Dose adjustment generally required for C_{cr} <70 ml/min/1.73m².

††This range applies to C_{cr} 6-20 ml/min/1.73m²; the upper range may be associated with increased risk of seizures. The drug should not be used when C_{cr} <5ml/min/1.73m² unless the patient is on hemodialysis.

‡‡50% standard dose recommended for GFR ≤30 ml/min.

§§If C_{cr} ≥60ml/min.

‖‖If C_{cr} 21-60 ml/min.

***If C_{cr} <20 ml/min.

†††If C_{cr} 30-50 ml/min.

‡‡‡If C_{cr} 5-29 ml/min.

Antiparkinsonian drugs

Preparation	Average daily dose
Levodopa	1.5-8.0 g
Levodopa/carbidopa (Sinemet)	300-1200 mg
Levodopa/benserazide (Madopa)	300-1200 mg
Amantadine (Symmetrel)	100-300 mg
Trihexyphenidyl (Artane)	2-15 mg
Benztropine (Cogentin)	1.0-6.0 mg
Ethopropazide (Parsidol)	100-400 mg
Bromocriptine (Parlodel)	7.5-30 mg (with DOPA)
Pergolide (Permax)	1.5-4.0 mg
Selegeline (Eldepryl)	5-10 mg

Antiparkinsonian agents

Properties of various beta-adrenergic blocking agents

Agent	Cardioselectivity	Intrinsic sympathetic activity	Lipid solubility	Plasma half-life (hours)	Usual dose for angina
Propranolol	–	–	+++	1-6	60-320 mg/day
Metoprolol	+	–	+	3	100-200 mg/day
Nadolol	–	–	0	16-24	80-240 mg/day
Timolol	–	–	+	4-5	15-45 mg/day
Atenolol	+	–	0	6-9	50-100 mg/day
Pindolol	–	+++	+	4	5-20 mg/day
Acebutolol	+	++	0	8-12	600-1200 mg/day
Labetolol (combined beta- or alpha-blocking effects)	–	–	+++	3-4	300-600 mg/day

Calcium channel blocking agents potentially useful in management of angina syndromes

Agent	Usual dose	Absolute or relative contraindications
Dihydropyridines		
Nifedipine	Oral: 30–120 mg/day Sublingual: 10 mg q4–6 h	Hypotension
Nitrendipine	20–40 mg/day	Hypotension
Felodipine (potent vasodilator)	15–30 mg/day	Hypotension
Nimodipine (useful in cerebral ischemia)	0–35 mg/kg, 4 hourly	Hypotension
Nisoldipine	30–60 mg/day	Hypotension
Nicardipine	15–90 mg/day	Hypotension
Verapamil	IV bolus: 5–10 mg in 10 min IV infusion: 1 mg/min to total of 10 mg Oral: 120–480 mg/day	Sick sinus syndrome, A-V conduction defects, sinus bradycardia, digitalis toxicity, overt heart failure, hypotension
Diltiazem	IV: 0.15–0.25 mg/kg over 2 min Oral: 90–230 mg/day	As for verapamil
Mixed agents		
Tiapamil (as with verapamil, also a sodium blocker)	1500 mg/day	As for verapamil
Bepridil (mixed sodium blocker)	200–400 mg/day	Prolonged Q-T interval

Drugs used in treatment of cancer

Drug	Route of administration	Acute toxicity
I. *Alkylating agents*. The alkyl group of these molecules forms covalent bonds with DNA and thus interferes with its replication. This interference not only is cytotoxic, but also is potentially mutagenic and carcinogenic		
A. Mustard derivatives		
Mechlorethamine, nitrogen mustard (Mustargen)	IV, Intrapleural	Nausea and vomiting, local phlebitis; chemical cellulitis and tissue necrosis if drug extravasates
Cyclophosphamide† (Cytoxan), ifosfamide (IFEX)	IV, oral	Nausea and vomiting with intermittent high dose
Chlorambucil (Leukeran)	Oral	Daily doses well tolerated; may be slight nausea and vomiting
Melphalan (Alkeran)	Oral, IV (experimental)	Daily doses well tolerated; may be slight nausea and vomiting
B. Alkyl sulfonate		
Busulfan (Myleran)	Oral	None
C. Ethylenimine		
triethylenethiophosphoramide (Thiotepa)	IV	None
D. Triazene		
Dacarbazine (DTIC)	IV	Nausea and vomiting that lessens with repetitive doses; occasional flulike syndrome; pain and tissue damage if extravasated

Intermediate or delayed toxicity*	Precautions
Bone marrow suppression; alopecia	Administer through a running IV infusion; must be given immediately on reconstitution because of short physical half-life.
Bone marrow suppression; chemical cystitis; alopecia; syndrome of inappropriate antidiuretic hormone (SIADH)	Use forced hydration to induce polyuria to avoid *cystitis* (metabolites of drug irritate the bladder). Mesna (see under miscellaneous) is administered with IFEX to prevent hemorrhagic cystitis.
Bone marrow suppression	None
Bone marrow suppression	None
Bone marrow suppression; *pulmonary fibrosis*, hyperpigmentation of skin, gynecomastia	None
Bone marrow suppression	None
Bone marrow suppression, hepatic toxicity	Avoid extravasation.

Continued.

Drugs used in treatment of cancer—cont'd

Drug	Route of administration	Acute toxicity
E. Nitrosoureas		
Carmustine (BiCNU)	IV	Burning pain along vein, facial flushing, nausea and vomiting within 4 to 6 hours
Lomustine (CeeNU)	Oral	Nausea and vomiting
Streptozocin (Za-nosar)	IV	Nausea and vomiting, renal tubular acidosis, renal failure
F. Platinum analogs		
Cisplatin (Platinol)	IV	Nausea and vomiting; mild bone marrow suppression
Carboplatin (Parapl-atin)	IV	Nausea and vomiting, bone marrow suppression, especially thrombocytopenia
G. Altretamine (Hexalen)	Oral	Mild nausea and vomiting, mild marrow suppression
II. *Antimetabolites*. Structural analogs of normal metabolites that compete with normal metabolites in the synthesis of RNA and/or DNA. This interferes with normal cellular replication.		
A. Folate analogs		
Methotrexate (MTX)	Oral, IV, SC, IM, IT	Nausea and vomiting with high doses

Intermediate or delayed toxicity*	Precautions
Bone marrow suppression 3 to 6 weeks after administration, occasional renal and hepatic toxicity	Slow infusion rate to prevent local pain; cumulative bone marrow suppression may occur.
As for carmustine	
Diabetes mellitus	Inject through running IV infusion; avoid extravasation.
High-frequency hearing loss, distal sensory neuropathy	Forced saline hydration can prevent renal damage; otherwise, irreversible renal failure may occur.
Thrombocytopenia, possibly cumulative	Dosage may be adjusted according to renal function.
Peripheral neuropathy	Avoid concurrent monoamine oxidase inhibitors.
Bone marrow suppression, stomatitis, vasculitis, "MTX lung," cirrhosis with long-term use	Measure blood urea nitrogen, creatinine; creatinine clearance *must* be measured before instituting therapy and periodically thereafter. Dosage adjustment is obligatory if the creatinine clearance is not normal. Saline hydration and $NaHCO_3$ administration to alkalinize the urine is indicated for doses of 3 g/m^2 or greater to prevent MTX crystalluria with consequent renal failure.

Continued.

Drugs used in treatment of cancer—cont'd

Drug	Route of administration	Acute toxicity
B. Purine analogs		
6-Mercaptopurine† (6-MP) (Puri-nethol)	Oral	Nausea and vomiting, anorexia rare
Thioguanine† (6-TG) (Tabloid)	Oral	Rare gastrointestinal intolerance
Fludarabine (Fludara)	IV	Bone marrow suppression
C. Pyrimidine analogs		
5-Fluorouracil† (5-FU)	IV	Occasional nausea and vomiting
Cytarabine,† cytosine arabinoside, arabinosylcytosine, ara-C (Cytosar)	IV, SC, IM, IT	Nausea and vomiting with intermediate or high doses; repetitive high doses possibly associated with central nervous system, hepatic, pulmonary, and skin toxicity
III. *Plant alkaloids.* Interfere with mitotic spindle of the cell.‡		
Vincristine (Oncovin)	IV	Severe inflammatory reaction from extravasated drug
Vinblastine (Velban)	IV	Inflammatory reaction from extravasated drug

Intermediate or delayed toxicity*	Precautions
Bone marrow suppression, rare hepatocellular toxicity	*Allopurinol* may prevent drug catabolism; therefore 6-MP dose should be reduced to two-thirds to one-third the usual dose if given with allopurinol.
Bone marrow suppression	None
High doses associated with central nervous system toxicity, coma, cortical blindness	None
Bone marrow suppression, stomatitis, cerebellar ataxia, diarrhea	Monthly loading regimens may be more toxic than weekly doses; accumulates in effusions; decrease dose with severe liver disease.
Bone marrow suppression	None
Loss of deep tendon reflexes; constipation; impotence; paresthesia; neurotoxicity, possibly leading to foot or wristdrop or cranial nerve palsies; alopecia; rare abdominal, chest, or jaw pain; bone marrow suppression minimal	Inject through running IV infusion; avoid extravasation.
Bone marrow suppression, alopecia, occasional mild peripheral neuropathy	Inject slowly into vein or through running IV infusion.

Continued.

Cancer chemotherapeutic agents—cont'd

Drugs used in treatment of cancer—cont'd

Drug	Route of administration	Acute toxicity
IV. *Epipodophyllotoxins*. Inhibit topoisomerase II, DNA-processing enzyme.		
VP-16-213, etoposide (VePesid)	IV, oral (50% bioavailability)	Occasional nausea and vomiting; hypotension with rapid IV injection; rare anaphylaxis
V. *Antibiotics*		
Dactinomycin, actinomycin D (Cosmegen)	IV	Severe inflammatory reaction from extravasated drug; nausea and vomiting, occasional cramps and diarrhea
Doxorubicin (Adriamycin)	IV	Severe inflammatory reaction from extravasated drug; local phlebitis, nausea and vomiting, red urine (drug)
Daunorubicin, daunomycin, rubidomycin (Cerubidine)	IV	Same as for doxorubicin
Mitoxantrone (Novantrone)	IV	Occasional nausea and vomiting; serum and urine with possible green tint

Intermediate or delayed toxicity*	Precautions
Bone marrow depression; leukopenia more prominent; alopecia; mild peripheral neuropathy (may be additive with vincristine); mild diarrhea; abnormal liver function tests	Infuse drug over 30 minutes or longer; cardiovascular precautions for hypotension.
Bone marrow suppression, stomatitis, diarrhea, erythema, hyperpigmentation with occasional desquamation in areas of previous irradiation, alopecia	Administer through running IV infusion.
Bone marrow suppression, alopecia, *radiation recall, cardiac toxicity* related to cumulative doses (>500-550 mg/m^2), stomatitis	Inject through running IV infusion. Use with caution in patients with history of heart disease. Monitor left ventricular ejection fraction. Intractable ventricular failure may occur and is dose related. Reduce dosage with renal or hepatic impairment.
Same as for doxorubicin except no radiation recall; *cardiotoxic* dose approximately 1000 mg/m^2	Same as for doxorubicin
Bone marrow depression; alopecia (less common than with anthracyclines); diarrhea; stomatitis; potential cardiotoxicity as function of cumulative dose; mild liver function test abnormality	Cardiac toxicity is function of *total cumulative* dose of *prior anthracyclines* plus dose of mitoxantrone. Drug precipitates with heparin.

Continued.

Drugs used in treatment of cancer—cont'd

Drug	Route of administration	Acute toxicity
Bleomycin (Blenoxane)	IV, IM, SC	Fever, chills, nausea and vomiting; immediate hypersensitivity in lymphoma patients
Mitomycin (Mutamycin)	IV	Nausea and vomiting; inflammatory reaction from extravasated drug
Mithramycin (Mithracin)	IV	
VI. *Miscellaneous*		
L-Asparaginase (Elspar)	IV, IM, SC	Immediate hypersensitivity reactions, fever, anorexia, nausea and vomiting
Procarbazine (Matulane)	Oral	Nausea and vomiting, especially if dose is escalated too rapidly; improves after first few days
Hydroxyurea (Hydrea)	Oral	Anorexia, nausea
Mesna (Mesnex)	IV	Nausea and vomiting, bad taste in mouth

Intermediate or delayed toxicity*	Precautions
Striae and hyperpigmentation of skin, sore or ulcerated fingertips, rash, alopecia; diffuse pulmonary interstitial infiltrate leading to irreversible *pulmonary fibrosis,* especially with cumulative doses of 400 mg or greater; toxic dose possibly lower with previous radiation to lung or presence of other pulmonary toxins (e.g., methotrexate)	Immediate hypersensitivity with first 1 to 2 doses in lymphoma patients; follow serial pulmonary function tests, especially diffusion capacity.
Bone marrow suppression, stomatitis, alopecia, skin ulceration	Administer through running IV infusion.
Bone marrow suppression, hepatotoxicity with reduced synthesis of clotting factors, nephrotoxicity, hypocalcemia	Low therapeutic index; a severe bleeding diathesis can occur and may be fatal.
Hepatic dysfunction, decreased synthesis of liver proteins (albumin, clotting factors), decreased synthesis of insulin with nonketotic hyperglycemia and coma, pancreatitis	Potential for *immediate hypersensitivity* reaction must be considered; IV line must be in place and epinephrine at bedside.
Bone marrow depression after 3 to 4 weeks, lethargy, drowsiness, fever, myalgia, arthralgia	Decrease dose in patients with hepatic, renal, or marrow dysfunction; synergism with central nervous system depressants (phenothiazine, barbiturates) may be seen, as well as *Antabuse-like reaction* with ethanol. Monoamine oxidase inhibitory activity sometimes occurs. Sympathomimetic drugs, cheese, and bananas should be avoided.
Bone marrow depression, megaloblastic anemia; stomatitis, diarrhea, and alopecia are less common	Decrease dose in patients with marrow and renal dysfunction.
	Incompatible with cisplatin; false-positive urinary ketone test may occur.

Continued.

Drugs used in treatment of cancer—cont'd

Drug	Route of administration	Acute toxicity
VII. *Steroids*		
Glucocorticoids	Oral, IV, IT	Epigastric distress
Estrogens	Oral	Nausea and vomiting with large doses; slow *escalation* of dose
Progestational agents	Oral, IM, SC	None
Androgens	Oral	Occasional nausea and vomiting more frequent at higher doses
Antiandrogen Flutamide (Eulexin)	Oral	Nausea and vomiting, hot flashes
Gonadotropin-releasing hormone agonist Leuprolide (Lupron)	SC, IM	Steroid flare, hot flashes
Aromatase inhibitor Aminoglutethimide (Cytadren)	Oral	Nausea and vomiting
VIII. *Biologic response modifiers*		
Interferon alpha-2a (Roferon-A)	IM, SC	Flulike symptoms
Lymphokine (interleukin-2)	IV	Capillary leak syndrome, flulike syndrome

*The teratogenic and abortifacient properties of most anticancer drugs must be kept in mind when treating women of childbearing age. Many anticancer drugs have been shown to be carcinogenic in laboratory animals.

†Inactive in this commercial form; must be metabolized in vivo to the active drug.

‡Plant alkaloids, epipodophyllotoxins, and antibiotics are typically referred to as *natural products,* that is, derived from nature.

IV, Intravenous; SC, subcutaneous; IM, intramuscular; IT, intrathecal; RNA, ribonucleic acid; DNA, deoxyribonucleic acid.

Intermediate or delayed toxicity*	Precautions
Weight gain, truncal obesity, striae, skin fragility, moon facies, euphoria and psychosis, peptic ulcers, osteoporosis; enhanced risk of infection, diabetes, and hypertension	Consider prophylaxis for tuberculosis in patient with history of or exposure to tuberculosis or with lymphomas; use antacids for gastric distress.
Gynecomastia in men, breast tenderness in women; *high doses* have been implicated in *increased cardiovascular deaths* in men with prostate cancer	*Steroid flare:* serum calcium levels can rise rapidly in breast cancer patients shortly after therapy is started, especially in those with bony disease; edema may occur with poor cardiac function.
Occasional liver function abnormalities, alopecia, and hypersensitivity reactions	Use with care in presence of liver dysfunction; may be teratogenic to fetus; increases risk of thromboemboli.
Fluid retention, virilization (increased facial hair, acne, deepening of voice, clitoral hypertrophy), hypercalcemia, liver function abnormalities with rare jaundice, increased red cell mass	Use with care in elderly patients with cardiac, liver, or renal disease with nephrotic syndrome. Acute hypercalcemia may occur in immobilized patients.
Gynecomastia, impotence	
Gynecomastia, impotence	
Hypoadrenalism	
None	
Anaphylaxis	

Insulin preparations

Selected clinical characteristics of insulin preparations

Onset of action	Insulin	Duration of action (h)		Peak effect (h)		Compatible mixed with
		Initial	Chronic use	Initial	Chronic use	
Rapid	Crystalline zinc (CZI, regular crystalline soluble actrapid)	6	16	2-3	5-6	All insulin preparations
	Semilente	12		3-6		Lente preparations
Intermediate	Neutral protamine (Isophane, NPH)	14-24	24	6-12	10-12	Regular insulin
	Globin	18		6-8		
	Lente	18-24	24	8-14	10-12	Regular insulin and semilente preparations
Long	Protamine zinc (PZI)	36		16-24		
	Ultralene	36		20-30		Regular insulin and semilente preparations

Nitrate and nitrite drugs used in treatment of angina

Drug	Dosage	Duration of action
Short acting		
Nitroglycerin, sublingual	0.15-1.2 mg	10-30 min
Isosorbide, sublingual	2.5-5.0 mg	10-60 min
Amyl nitrite, inhalant	0.18-0.3 ml	3-5 min
Long acting		
Nitroglycerin, oral sustained-action	6.5-13 mg/6-8 hr	6-8 hr
		3-6 hr
Nitroglycerin, 2% ointment	1/2-2 inches/4 hr	3-6 hr
Nitroglycerin, slow-release buccal	1-2 mg/4 hr	1 1/2-2 hr
Nitroglycerin, slow-release transcutaneous	10-25 mg/24 hr	24 hr or longer
Isosorbide dinitrate, sublingual	2.5-10 mg/2 hr	4-6 hr
Isosorbide dinitrate, oral	10-60 mg/4-6 hr	4-6 hr
Isosorbide dinitrate, chewable	5-10 mg/2-4 hr	2-3 hr
Pentaerythrityl tetranitrate	40 mg/6-8 hr	6-8 hr
Erythrityl tetranitrate	10-40 mg/6-8 hr	6-8 hr

Published with permission from Katzung BG and Chatterjee K: Basic and clinical pharmacology. Los Altos, Calif, 1983, Lange.

Nitroglycerin preparations

Some nonsteroidal anti-inflammatory drugs

Drug	Dose range (mg/day)	Half-life (h)	Side effects Dyspepsia, ulcer, etc.	Side effects Others
Short serum half-life				
Diclofenac	75-200	1	+ +	Hepatotoxicity
Etodolac	600-1200	6-7	+	—
Fenoprofen	1200-3200	2	+ +	Nephrotoxicity
Flurbiprofen	200-400	3-4	+	—
Ibuprofen	1200-3200	2	+ +	—
Ketoprofen	100-400	2	+ +	—
Ketorolac	60-150 I.M. 10-60 oral	4-6	+ +	—
Meclofenamate sodium	200-400	2-3	+ +	Diarrhea
Tolmetin	800-2000	1	+ +	—
Long serum half-life				
Indomethacin	50-200	3-11	+ + + +	Headache
Nabumetone	1000-2000	23-30	+	—
Naproxen	250-1500	13	+	—
Piroxicam	20	30-86	+ +	—
Sulindac	300-400	16	+ +	—
Oxaprozin	600-1800	21	+	—
Salicylate				
Aspirin	1000-6000	4-15	+ + + +	Tinnitus
Choline magnesium salicylate	1500-4000	4-15	+	Tinnitus
Salicyl salicylate	1500-5000	4-15	+	Tinnitus
Diflunisal	500-1500	7-15	+ +	—

Drugs used to treat patients with active peptic ulcers

Generic name	Trade name	Duodenal ulcer*		Gastric ulcer†	
		Dosages for adults (ml or mg/day)	Frequency of administration (times/day)	Dosages for adults (ml or mg/day)	Frequency of administration (times/day)
Drugs that inhibit acid secretion					
H$_2$-receptor antagonists					
Cimetidine	Tagamet	300 mg	With each meal and at bedtime (four times daily)	300 mg	With each meal and at bedtime (four times daily)
		400 mg	Twice daily, in the morning and at bedtime		
Ranitidine	Zantac	800 mg	Once daily at bedtime	800 mg	Once daily at bedtime
		150 mg	Twice daily, in the morning and at bedtime	150 mg	Twice daily, in the morning and at bedtime
		300 mg	Once daily at bedtime		
Famotidine	Pepcid	40 mg	Once daily at bedtime	40 mg	Once daily at bedtime
Nizatidine	Axid	300 mg	Once daily at bedtime	‡	‡
Proton pump inhibitors Omeprazole	Prilosec	20 mg	Once daily	‡	‡
Drugs that coat the ulcer crater Sucralfate	Carafate	1 g	Four times daily	‡	‡

*Most patients with duodenal ulcers are treated for 4-6 weeks.
†Most patients with gastric ulcers are treated for 8-12 weeks.
‡Not approved by U.S. Food and Drug Administration.

Characteristics of oral hypoglycemic agents (sulfonylureas)

Generic name	Brand name	Strength (mg)	Onset of action (hr)	Duration of action (hr)	Dosage range (mg)	Major toxicity
Tolbutamide	Orinase	500	0.5	6–12	500–3000	Photosensitivity after alcohol ingestion; occasionally hypoglycemia
Chlorpropamide	Diabinese	100, 250	1	60–90	100–500	Hypersensitivity, jaundice, skin rash, pancytopenia; occasionally edema, hypo-natremia
Acetohexamide	Dymelor	250, 500	0.5	12–24	250–1500	Hypoglycemia, gastrointestinal disturbances, head-ache; occasionally allergic skin manifestations, photosensitivity, jaundice
Tolazamide	Tolinase	100, 250, 500	4–6	10–18	100–1000	Rare gastrointestinal disturbances
Glyburide	Micronase	1.25, 2.5, 5	1	18–24	2.5–20.0	Hypoglycemia
Glipizide	Glucotrol	5, 10	0.5	12–24	5–40	Hypoglycemia

Laboratory Evaluation

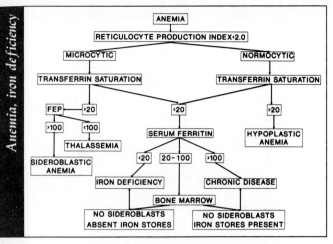

A rational approach to the laboratory diagnosis of iron deficiency anemia and the other common disorders that must be considered in the differential diagnosis.

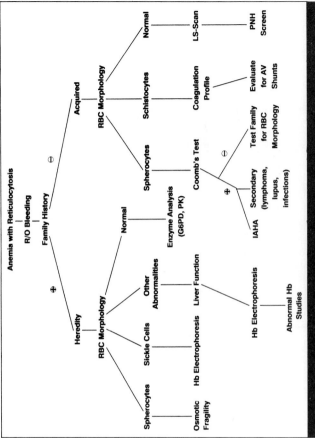

Evaluations of patients with hemolytic anemia. *LS,* liver spleen; *AV,* arteriovenous; *PNH,* paroxysmal nocturnal hemoglobinuria; *IAHA,* idiopathic autoimmune hemolytic anemia; *Hb,* hemoglobin.

ANA specificities and disease associations

Antibody to	Disease association
1. Double-stranded (native) DNA	Highly specific for SLE (40%-60% incidence) when in moderate to high titer
2. Single-stranded (denatured) DNA	Present in SLE and other rheumatic and nonrheumatic diseases
3. Individual histones, H1, H2A, H2B, H3, H4	SLE (70%) drug-induced LE (>95%), RA (15%)
4. Histone complexes H2A-H2B	Drug-induced LE (>60%)
5. Sm (proteins complexed with U-RNAs)	SLE (30%), highly specific
6. U1-RNP (proteins complexed with U1-RNA)	MCTD (>95%), SLE (35%)
7. SS-A/Ro (proteins with small RNAs)	SS (70%), SLE (50%), other CTDs
8. SS-B/La (45K protein with RNA polymerase III transcripts)	SS (40%-50%), SLE (15%)
9. Proliferating cell nuclear antigen (PCNA/cyclin)	SLE (3%)
10. Ma antigen	SLE (20%)
11. Ki antigen	SLE (12%)
12. Scl-70 (topoisomerase I)	PSS (20%) highly specific
13. Centromere/kinetochore	CREST (70%-90%), diffuse scleroderma (10%-20%)
14. RANA (rheumatoid arthritis–associated nuclear antigen [EBV related])	RA (90%)
15. Mi-1	Dermatomyositis (11%)
16. Jo-1 (histidyl-tRNA synthetase)	Polymyositis (31%)
17. Ku	Polymyositis-scleroderma overlap (55%)
18. NuMa (nuclear mitotic apparatus) antigen	RA, Sjögren's syndrome, carpal tunnel syndrome
19. PM/Scl (PM-1)	Polymyositis-scleroderma overlap

EBV, Epstein-Barr virus; SLE, systemic lupus erythematosus; MCTD, mixed connective tissue disease; SS, Sjögren's syndrome; PSS, progressive systemic sclerosis; CREST, calcinosis, Raynaud's phenomenon, esophageal hypomotility, sclerodactyly, and telangiectasia; RA, rheumatoid arthritis.

A diagram for the laboratory evaluation of a patient with a bleeding disorder in whom the history and physical examination suggest an acquired coagulation disorder

	PTT	PT	TT	Inh	FDP	Plt
Liver disease						
Acute hepatitis, early liver disease		A				
Chronic liver disease	A	A	A	A	A	A
Disseminated intravascular coagulation (DIC)	A	A	A	A	A	A
Vitamin K deficiency, warfarin ingestion	A	A				
Heparin administration	A	A	A	A		
Lupus anticoagulant	A	A*		A		
Acquired factor VIII inhibitor	A			A		

PTT, Partial thromboplastin time; PT, prothrombin time; TT, thrombin time; Inh, coagulation inhibitor screening test; FDP, fibrin degradation products; Plt, platelet count; A, abnormal result; A*, often the PT is abnormal only when dilute thromboplastin is used.

Bleeding disorder, acquired

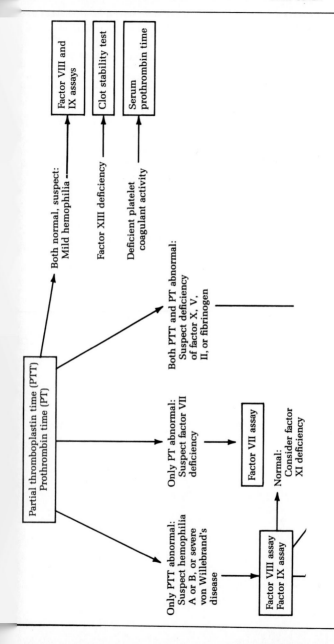

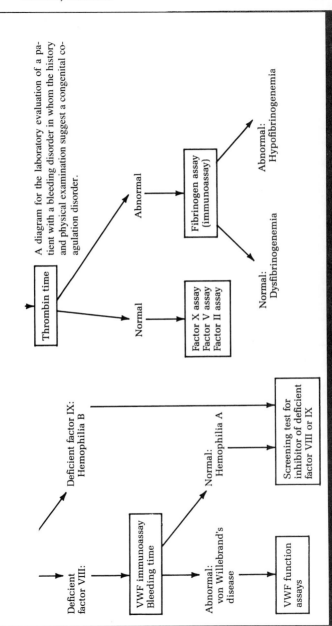

A diagram for the laboratory evaluation of a patient with a bleeding disorder in whom the history and physical examination suggest a congenital coagulation disorder.

Thrombin time

Abnormal → Fibrinogen assay (immunoassay)

Normal → Factor X assay / Factor V assay / Factor II assay

Abnormal: Hypofibrinogenemia

Normal: Dysfibrinogenemia

Deficient factor IX: Hemophilia B

Deficient factor VIII:

VWF immunoassay / Bleeding time

Normal: Hemophilia A → Screening test for inhibitor of deficient factor VIII or IX

Abnormal: von Willebrand's disease → VWF function assays

Bleeding disorder, congenital coagulation abnormality

Diagnostic tests useful in fever and rash

Test	Application
Aspirate of lesion for Gram stain and culture	Most helpful in pustular or petechial lesions. Positive in up to 60% of meningococcemias
Wright or Giemsa stain of vesicular fluid	Up to 70% of herpesvirus infections will show multinucleated giant cells or cytoplasmic inclusion bodies
Biopsy	Fungal infections, vasculitis, granulomatous disease Immunofluorescence: RMSF, SLE
Cultures of distant sites	
Blood	All cases of possible bacteremia, fungemia
Throat, rectal swab	Viral infections
Throat, rectum, urethra, cervix, joint	Disseminated gonococcal infection
Serologic testing	Streptococcal and rickettsial infections, syphilis, typhoid fever, leptospirosis, Lyme disease (*B. burgdorferi* spirochete), *Mycoplasma,* coccidioidomycosis, hepatitis B, Epstein-Barr virus, cytomegalovirus, measles, atypical measles, SLE, trichinosis, enterovirus and adenovirus infections

Fever and rash

Serologic tests for diagnosis of fungal disease

Disease	Test	Comment
Histoplasmosis	Complement fixation	Titer <1:8 is nonspecific.
	Immunodiffusion complement fixation	May be negative in up to one third of disseminated histoplasmosis patients. Tends to level off at 1:32 maximum titer, though may be higher. With yeast phase antigen, is higher in disease. With mycelial antigen, may be boosted by positive skin test to histoplasmin. Extensive cross-reaction with *B. dermatitidis*. Low-grade cross-reaction with *C. immitis*.
	Immunodiffusion	H band and M bands are specific, and one or both are positive in up to 90% of patients.
	Radioimmunoassay for antigen	Investigational in serum and urine. Highly useful in rapid diagnosis and monitoring treatment response in disseminated histoplasmosis. Available from Dr. J. Wheat, University of Indiana, Indianapolis.
Coccidioidomycosis	Complement fixation or immunodiffusion complement fixation	Specific, with only minimal cross-reaction in histoplasmosis. Highest titers occur in most severely ill patients (titer $\geq 1:6$ associated with serious disease). Titer rises more slowly and is more sustained than in the precipitin test. Any titer in cerebrospinal fluid is diagnostic of meningitis. May be used to follow the course of disease; that is a declining titer is a good prognostic sign.
	Tube precipitin or immunodiffusion tube precipitin	Highly specific. Converts to positive in over 85% of patients, usually within weeks of infection. Cannot be titrated. Usually reverts to negative quickly, even though active disease persists.

Disease	Test	Comment
Blastomycosis	Radioimmunoassay for antigen	Investigational (J. Galgiani, University of Arizona, Tucson).
	Complement fixation	Positive in only 50%-70% of patients. Highly cross-reactive with *H. capsulatum*.
Paracoccidioidomycosis	Immunodiffusion for bands 1 and 2	Specific, but is not titrated. Not helpful in assessing activity of disease.
	Complement fixation	As in coccidioidomycosis, higher titers occur with more severe disease. Cross-reacts with *H. capsulatum*.
Sporotrichosis	Complement fixation	No widespread serologic tests.
Aspergillosis	Immunodiffusion	Helpful in confirming diagnosis of allergic bronchopulmonary and mycetoma forms. Often negative in widespread dissemination.
	Immunoassay for circulating antigen	Specific but not sensitive. May be useful in disseminated disease. Investigational and not widely available. (V. Andriole, Yale University, New Haven, Conn.).
Candidiasis	Immunodiffusion	Antibodies present in many normal persons. Not especially helpful in diagnosis of disease.
	Multiple-antigen tests	Variable in sensitivity and specificity for *Candida* antigen and intermittently promising. None have survived beyond initial efforts at marketing. The lack of *Candida* and *Aspergillus* antigen testing is a great impediment to rapid diagnosis of mycosis in the leukopenic host and is a primary driving force perpetuating empiric use of antifungal agents.
Zygomycosis	No serologic tests available	
Nocardiosis	No serologic tests available	
Actinomycosis	No serologic tests available	
Chromomycosis	No serologic tests available	
Phaeohyphomycosis	No serologic tests available	
Fusarium	No serologic tests available	
Trichosporonosis	No serologic tests available	May see a "false positive" test for cryptococcal capsulatum polysaccharide.

Peripheral blood morphology (Wright's stained smears) as a guide to evaluation of patients with suspected hemolytic disease

Blood smear findings	Differential diagnosis		Further tests (in order of priority)
	Congenital	Acquired	
Spherocytes	HS, Hb CC	Immune, burns	Direct Coombs, osm. fragil., Hb electrophoresis
Elliptocytes, poikilocytes	HE, HPP	Myelodysplasia	Osm. fragil., specialized membrane studies
Hypochromic microcytes, "leptocytes"	Thalassemia, Hb Lepore, sideroblast	Iron defic., lead poisoning sideroblast	Fe/TIBC, Hb A_2 and F, Hb electrophoresis, marrow, DNA probes
Sickle cells	SS, SA, SC		Hb electrophoresis
Target cells (normocytic)	AC, SC, CC	—	Hb electrophoresis
Acanthocytes	PK defic., abetalipoproteinemia	Obstructive jaundice, post splenectomy	PK screen, LFTs, lipid panel
Stomatocytes	Hydro-cytosis or xerocytosis, Rh null	Liver disease	Red cell Na/K and water content
		Liver disease, alcohol	

Erythrophagocytosis, clumped RBC	Immune	—	Direct Coombs, D-L test, cold agglutinins
Schistocytes	TTP, DIC, heart valve defects, myelodysplasia	Kasabach-Merritt syndrome	Cardiac auscultation, coagulation tests
Blister cells, eccentrocytes	Oxidant poisoning	G6PD defic., unstable Hb pyr-5'-nucleot. defic.	G6PD screen, test for unstable Hb
Heavy basophilic stippling	Lead poisoning		Lead screen, specialized enzyme assay
Nondescript or no changes	PNH, internal bleeding†, recovering marrow†	G6PD, most glycolytic defects	Sucrose lysis test, acid lysis test, G6PD screen, PK screen, specialized enzyme assays

†These conditions may simulate hemolytic disease because both feature the combination of anemia and a high reticulocyte count.

HS, hereditary spherocytosis; HE, hereditary elliptocytosis; HPP, hereditary pyropoikilocytosis; osm. fragil., osmotic fragility; sideroblast., sideroblastic anemia; Hb, hemoglobin; SS, SA, SC, CC, A_2, F, hemoglobin variants; Fe/TIBC, iron and iron-binding capacity; PK, pyruvate kinase; defic., deficiency; LFTs, liver function tests; D-L test, Donath-Landsteiner test; TTP, thrombotic thrombocytopenic purpura; DIC, disseminated intravascular coagulation; G6PD, glucose-6-phosphate dehydrogenase; pyr'5'-nucleot, pyrimidine-5'-nucleotidase; PNH, paroxysmal nocturnal hemoglobinuria; Rh null, congenital absence of Rh antigens.

Liver function test patterns in hepatobiliary disorders and jaundice

Type of disorder	Bilirubin	Aminotransferases
Hemolysis Gilbert's syndrome	Normal to 5 mg/dl 85% due to indirect fractions No bilirubinuria	Normal
Acute hepatocellular necrosis (viral and drug hepatitis, hepatotoxins, acute heart failure)	Both fractions may be elevated Peak usually follows aminotransferases Bilirubinuria	Elevated, often >500 IU ALT ≥ AST
Chronic hepatocellular disorders	Both fractions may be elevated Bilirubinuria	Elevated, but usually <300 IU
Alcoholic hepatitis Cirrhosis	Both fractions may be elevated Bilirubinuria	AST/ALT >2 suggests alcoholic hepatitis or cirrhosis
Intrahepatic cholestasis Obstructive jaundice	Both fractions may be elevated Bilirubinuria	Normal to moderate elevation Rarely >500 IU
Infiltrative diseases (tumor, granulomata); partial bile duct obstruction	Usually normal	Normal to slight elevation

Alkaline phosphatase	Albumin	Globulin	Prothrombin time
Normal	Normal	Normal	Normal
Normal to <3 times normal elevation	Normal	Normal	Usually normal. If >5s above control and not corrected by parenteral vitamin K, suggests poor prognosis
Normal to <3 times normal elevation	Often decreased	Increased gamma globulin	Often prolonged Fails to correct with parenteral vitamin K
Normal to <3 times normal elevation	Often decreased	Increased IGA and increased gamma globulin	
Elevated, often >4 times normal elevation	Normal, unless chronic	Gamma globulin normal Beta globulin may be increased	Normal If prolonged, will correct with parenteral vitamin K
Elevated, often >4 times normal elevation Fractionate, or confirm liver origin with 5'-nucleotidase, gamma glutamyl transpeptidase	Normal	Usually normal Gamma globulin may be increased in granulomatous disease	Normal

Useful laboratory tests in evaluation of intestinal malabsorption

Test	Impaired intraluminal digestion	Mucosal disease	Lymphatic obstruction	Limitations
Stool fat (qualitative, quantitative)	Increased (concentration usually >9.5%)	Increased (concentration usually <9.5%)	Increased	False-negative result if inadequate ingestion of dietary fat or recent barium ingestion; false-positive result with castor oil or mineral oil ingestion
Serum carotene	Decreased	Decreased	Decreased	Low values may occur in normal subjects who ingest little dietary carotene
Serum cholesterol	Decreased	Decreased	Decreased	May be normal or increased in patients with untreated lipoprotein abnormality
Serum albumin	Usually normal, except with bacterial overgrowth	Often decreased	Often decreased	
Prothrombin activity	Decreased if severe	Decreased if severe	Decreased if severe	May also be decreased in liver disease, but parenterally administered vitamin K should induce normalization if caused by malabsorption

Test				
Serum iron	Normal	Often decreased	Normal	
Serum folate	Normal	Often decreased	Normal	
Xylose absorption	Normal, except with bacterial overgrowth	Abnormal, unless disease confined to distal small intestine	Normal	Requires normal gastric emptying and renal function
Lactose absorption (lactose tolerance test or breath hydrogen after lactose load)	Normal, except in some instances of bacterial overgrowth	Increase in plasma glucose <20 mg/dl; increased breath H_2	Normal	May be abnormal in all categories if patient has primary intestinal lactase deficiency
Vitamin B_{12} (Schilling test)	Decreased in bacterial overgrowth and exocrine pancreatic insufficiency	Decreased in extensive ileal disease	Normal	Requires good renal function
^{14}C-cholylglycine breath tests	Increased $^{14}CO_2$ excretion in bacterial overgrowth	Increased $^{14}CO_2$ excretion in ileal disease	Normal	Requires normal gastric emptying
Lactulose breath test	Early appearance of H_2 in breath in bacterial overgrowth	Normal	Normal	Requires normal gastric emptying; false-positive results may occur in patient with rapid small intestinal transit
Secretin/cholecystokinin stimulation tests	Abnormal in chronic pancreatic disease	Normal	Normal	Relatively low sensitivity
Peroral intestinal biopsy	Normal except in severe bacterial overgrowth	Often abnormal	Often abnormal	May miss patchy mucosal disease

Typical CSF findings in acute meningitis

Test	Bacterial meningitis	Aseptic meningitis syndrome
Cell count	<100->10,000, usually 1000-5000	<10->1000, usually 100-500
Percentage of granulo-cytes	≥80	≤50*
Protein	100-500, occasionally >1000	100-500
Glucose	≤40	Normal†
Gram stain	Positive 75%-80%	Negative‡
Culture	Positive 70%-85%	Negative§
Acid-fast stain	Negative	Positive in tuberculosis (15%->60%)
India ink	Negative	Positive in cryptococcal disease (50%-75%)
Cytology	Negative	Positive in cryptococcal or neoplastic (≥70%) disease
Wet mount	Usually negative	Positive in amebic meningitis
Counterimmunoelectro-phoresis	Positive‖	Negative
Lactate	Positive (≥35 mg/dl)	Negative
Limulus lysate	Positive**	Negative
Cryptococcal antigen	Negative	Positive in cryptococcal (≥95%) disease
Enzymes (e.g., lactate dehydrogenase)	Often elevated	Often elevated
Cyclic adenosine mono-phosphate	Decreased	Unknown
Adenosine deaminase	Negative	Positive in tuberculosis (≥80%)
C-reactive protein	Positive	Negative

*May be ≥50% in early tuberculous, fungal, amebic, spirochetal, or viral meningitis.

†Commonly, CSF glucose is low in meningitis due to *M. tuberculosis, C. neoformans,* and other fungi; neoplasia; chemicals; sarcoidosis (~10%); syphilis (50%-55%); and sub-arachnoid hemorrhage. It is under 40 mg/dl in less than 5% of viral cases (especially mumps and LCM).

‡May be positive in fungal meningitis (e.g., 40% with *Candida* sp.).

§Positive in tuberculous (≥80%) and cryptococcal (50%) meningitis, and, rarely, in viral syndromes.

‖Positive response rates on CIE, staphylococcal coagglutination, and latex agglutination vary with infecting organisms (see text).

**The *Limulus* lysate test is positive only in gram-negative meningitis (≥90%).

Tests of pancreatic exocrine function

I. Direct-stimulation tests
- A. Secretin tests
  1. Submaximal secretin test (single IV injection, 1 CU/kg)
  2. Maximum secretin test
     - a. Single injection (2-4 CU/kg)
     - b. Continuous IV infusion (2-4 CU/kg/h)
  3. Augmented secretin test, bolus IV (1 CU/kg, then repeated with 4 CU/kg IV)
- B. Cholecystokinin (CCK)
  1. Single IV injection (3 CHR U/kg)
  2. Continuous IV injection (0.25 CHR U/kg/min)
- C. Combination of secretin and CCK tests
  1. Single injection
  2. Continuous IV infusion

II. Indirect-stimulation tests
- A. Lundh test meal
- B. ^{75}Se test meal, modification of Lundh test meal
- C. Duodenal perfusion of
  1. Essential amino acids
  2. Fatty acids
  3. Hydrochloric acid
- D. Synthetic peptide BZ-ty-PABA

III. Fecal tests
- A. Quantitative fecal fat and nitrogen
- B. Fecal excretion of ^{131}I-labeled triolein
- C. Fecal staining for fat
- D. Fecal examination for meat fibers
- E. Fecal enzyme determination

IV. Absorption tests
- A. ^{131}I-labeled triolein
- B. ^{131}I-labeled triolein and oleic acid
- C. Gelatin
- D. Starch
- E. Glucose

Pancreatic exocrine function

Pleural fluid classification

	Transudate	Exudate
Pleural TP/Serum TP	<0.5	>0.5
LDH	<2/3 upper normal limit	>2/3 upper normal limit
Pleural LDH/Serum LDH	<0.6	>0.6
WBC	<1000	>1000
RBC	<1000	>100,000
Glucose	=blood	<blood

TP, total protein; LDH, lactic dehydrogenase; WBC, white blood count; RBC, red blood count.

Classification of synovial effusions

Gross examination	Normal	"Noninflammatory"	Inflammatory	Septic
Viscosity	High	High	Low	Variable
Color	Colorless to straw-colored	Straw-colored to yellow	Yellow	Variable
Clarity	Transparent	Transparent	Cloudy	Opaque
WBC (per mm^3)	<200	200 to 2000	2000 to 75,000	Often >100,000
PMN leukocytes (%)	<25	<25	Often >50	>75
Mucin clot	Firm	Firm	Friable	Friable
Glucose (A.M. fasting)	Nearly equal to blood	Nearly equal to blood	<25 mg/dl lower than in blood	>25 mg/dl lower than in blood

Tumor markers

General uses:

1. Monitor serial titers before and after therapy. For example, a high preoperative CEA titer that falls to the normal range postoperatively is associated with a better prognosis in breast or colon cancer than is one that remains elevated after local therapy.

2. Serial values are also of use in monitoring (a) the clinical course of disease after local therapy and (b) the response to systemic chemotherapy. A decline in elevated values is usually consistent with tumor regression. Tumor markers are most valuable in monitoring disease not readily assessable by physical examination or simple radiographs.

	Characteristics	Presence in normal serum/plasma	Conditions in which elevated serum/plasma concentrations occur	
			Neoplastic	Nonneoplastic
I. Oncofetal proteins				
1. Carcinoembryonic antigen (CEA)	Glycoprotein (MW 200,000)	<2.5 ng/ml	Gastrointestinal, breast, lung cancers	Inflammatory bowel disease, pancreatitis, gastritis, smoker's chronic bronchitis, alcoholic liver disease, hepatitis
2. Alpha fetoprotein (AFP)	Alpha globulin (MW 70,000)	<40 ng/ml	Hepatoma, nonseminomatous testicular cancers	Pregnancy, regenerating liver tissue after viral hepatitis, chemically induced liver necrosis, partial hepatectomy

II. Hormones				
1. Human chorionic gonadotropin, beta subunit (β-HCG)	Glycoprotein (MW 45,000); beta subunit provides specificity versus LH, FSH, TSH	0	Choriocarcinoma, nonseminomatous testicular cancer, giant cell carcinoma of lung	Pregnancy
2. Ectopic hormones	ACTH, ADH, PTH		Lung, breast, head and neck, cervical cancers	
III. Serum enzymes				
1. Prostatic acid phosphatase (PAP)	Radioimmunoassay detects prostatic isozyme and distinguishes it from acid phosphatases of other organs (e.g., liver, spleen, kidney, small intestine), red and white blood cells, and platelets	0	Prostatic carcinoma	
2. Placental alkaline phosphatase	Biochemically and immunologically similar to that produced by the placenta	0	Seminoma, ovarian cancer	Pregnancy
3. Lactic dehydrogenase (LDH)	Tetramer, two distinct polypeptide chains: H (heart) and M (muscle)		Lymphoma	Hepatitis, myocardial infarction, muscle injury

Tumor markers—cont'd

	Characteristics	Presence in normal serum/plasma	Conditions in which elevated serum/plasma concentrations occur	
			Neoplastic	Nonneoplastic
IV. Immunoglobulins	Monoclonal elevation (M spike) of complete protein, light or heavy chain, or portions		Multiple myeloma, B cell lymphoma	Monoclonal gammopathy of unknown significance (M-GUS)
V. Tumor-associated antigens				
1. CA-125			Ovarian, lung cancers	Benign gynecologic disease, cirrhosis
2. CA-15.3			Breast, ovarian, lung cancers	
3. Prostate specific antigen	Glycoprotein (MW 30,000-40,000)		Prostatic carcinoma	Benign prostatic hypertrophy

MW, Molecular weight; LH, luteinizing hormone; FSH, follicle-stimulating hormone; TSH, thyroid-stimulating hormone; ACTH, adrenocorticotropic hormone; ADH, antidiuretic hormone; PTH, parathormone (parathyroid hormone).

Appendix

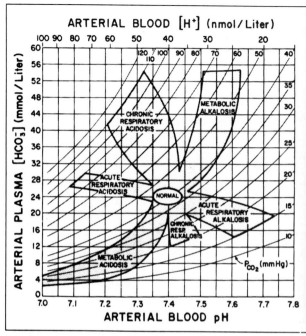

Acid-base nomogram. (Modified from Cogan MG and Rector FC Jr: Acid-base disorders. In Brenner BM and Rector FC Jr, editors: The kidney, Philadelphia, 1986, WB Saunders.)

Body surface area determination

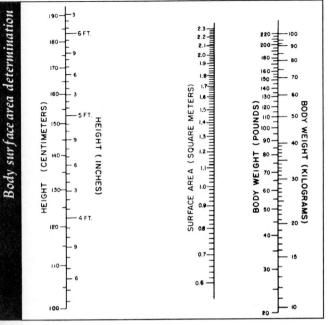

Nomogram for determining body surface area from height and weight. To determine body surface area from height *(left-hand scale)* and weight *(right-hand scale)*, these points are connected with a straightedge and surface area is read from the middle scale. (From Wilmore DW: The metabolic management of the critically ill. New York, 1977, Plenum Medical.)

Criteria for brain death in adults*

I. Cessation of all function of the entire brain
 A. Unresponsive coma
 B. Absent brainstem reflexes
  1. Pupillary light reflex
  2. Corneal reflex
  3. Cephalic (caloric) reflexes
  4. Oropharyngeal (gag) reflex
  5. Respiration (apnea testing)
II. Irreversibility
 A. Coma of known cause without potential for reversibility
 B. Exclusion of contributory, reversible conditions
  1. Drug intoxication
  2. Neuromuscular blockade
  3. Hypothermia (<32.2° C, 90°F)
  4. Shock
  5. Major metabolic disturbance
 C. Persistence for an appropriate period of observation (6-24 hours, depending on cause of coma and local practice)
III. Confirmatory investigations (may be optional or required)
 A. Electrocerebral silence (isoelectric EEG)
 B. Absence of circulation to the brain

Adapted and abridged from Guidelines for the determination of death: report of the medical consultants on the diagnosis of death to the President's Commission for the Study of Ethical Problems in Medicine and Biomedical and Behavioral Research. JAMA 246:2184, 1981.

*Note: Local and institutional rules are superseding.

Brain death criteria

Endocarditis prophylaxis regimen

Recommended prophylactic antibiotic regimens for patients at risk having dental, oral, upper respiratory tract, genitourinary, or gastrointestinal procedures

Procedure	Risk factor	Dosing regimen*	Comments
Dental, oral, or upper respiratory tract	Standard risk† with native valve	**Amoxicillin** 3 g orally 1 hr before procedure, then 1.5 g after initial dose.	Standard oral regimen
		Erythromycin 1 g orally 2 hr before procedure, then 0.5 g 6 hr after initial dose.	Amoxicillin/penicillin allergy.
		Clindamycin 300 mg orally 1 hr before procedure, then 150 mg 6 hr after initial dose.	Amoxicillin/penicillin allergy or unable to tolerate erythromycin.
		Ampicillin 2 g IV or IM 30 min before procedure, then 1 g IV or IM 6 hr after initial dose.	Unable to take oral medications.
		Clindamycin 300 mg IV 30 min before procedure, then 150 mg 6 hr after initial dose.	Unable to take oral medications; amoxicillin/ ampicillin/penicillin allergy.
	High risk† (prosthetic valve or history of endocarditis)	**Ampicillin** 2 g IV or IM plus **gentamicin** 1.5 mg/kg (not to exceed 80 mg) IV or IM 30 min before procedure, then amoxicillin 1.5 g orally 6 hr after initial dose.	Alternatively, instead of amoxicillin the IV regimen can be repeated 8 h after initial dose.

Genitourinary or gastrointestinal	Standard or high risk	**Vancomycin** 1 g IV starting 1 hr before procedure.	Amoxicillin/ampicillin/penicillin allergy; no repeat dose necessary.
		Ampicillin 2 g IV or IM plus **gentamicin** 1.5 mg/kg (not to exceed 80 mg) IV or IM 30 min before procedure, then amoxicillin 1.5 g orally 6 hr after initial dose.	Alternatively instead of oral amoxicillin the IV regimen can be repeated 8 hr after initial dose.
		Vancomycin 1 g IV plus **gentamicin** 1.5 mg/kg (not to exceed 80 mg) IV or IM starting 1 hr before procedure. May repeat gentamicin 8 hr after initial dose.	Amoxicillin/ampicillin/penicillin allergy; no repeat dose necessary for vancomycin.
	Low risk (minor procedures)‡	**Amoxicillin** 3 g orally 1 hr before procedure, then 1.5 g after initial dose.	Not for amoxicillin/penicillin-allergic patients.

Modified from Dajani AS et al: Prevention of bacterial endocarditis: recommendations by the American Heart Association. JAMA, 264:2919, 1990. Reader should refer to article for more detailed discussion of this topic.

*In patients with impaired renal function it may be necessary to omit second dose of gentamicin.

†Standard oral regimens can be used in higher risk patients as per AHA recommendations, however, clinicians may choose parenteral regimens.

‡Patients without prosthetic valve and no history of endocarditis and no urinary tract infection undergoing minor procedures.

Endocarditis prophylaxis regimen

Glasgow Coma Scale

Function tested	Response	Grade
1. Eye opening (E)	Spontaneously	E4
	To voice	3
	To pain	2
	None	1
C = eyes closed by swelling		
2. Best motor response	Obeys commands	M6
	Localizes pain	5
	Withdraws	4
	Decorticate to pain	3
	Decerebrate to pain	2
	None	1
3. Best verbal response	Oriented, appropriate	V5
	Confused conversation	4
	Inappropriate words	3
	Incomprehensible sounds	2
	None	1
T = intubated or tracheostomy		

Active and passive immunization against viral hepatitis

Virus	Exposure	Gamma globulin*		Vaccine*		Comments
		Dose	Timing	Recommen-dation	Timing	
A	Travel to endemic area	0.05 ml ISG/kg†	Repeat every 4-6 months	Yes	Vaccine should be available in United States in 1993 or 1994	0.02 ml ISG/kg sufficient for short visits
	Sexual or familial contact	0.02 ml ISG/kg	Within 7-14 days of exposure	Yes	—	
	Social or occupational contact	—	—	Yes	—	No prophylaxis recommended
B	Needle-stick or mucosal exposure	0.06 ml HBIG/kg†	Within 7 days of exposure	Yes	Immediately and at 1 and 6 months‡	Not necessary if recipient is HBsAg or anti-HBs positive
	Perinatal exposure to HBsAg (+) mother	0.50 ml HBIG	Single dose within 12 hours of birth	Yes	Within 12 hours of birth and at 1 and 6 months	HBIG and vaccine administered at separate sites

Hepatitis viral, immunizations

Sexual or close personal contact with patient with acute HB	0.06 ml HBIG/kg	Single dose	—	No	Vaccine recommended if expect continued exposure to patient with chronic HB
Familial or social contact with patient with acute HB	—	—	—		No prophylaxis recommended; vaccine recommended for young children of chronic carrier parent
C	Needle-stick or sexual exposure to hepatitis C	0.05 ml ISG/kg	Single dose	—	Generally recommended, although documentation of effectiveness is lacking

*Average dose is provided. Dosage of HBIG depends on titer of anti-HBs and should be in accordance with manufacturer's recommendations. Heptavax (plasma derived) and Recombivax and Engerix B (recombinant vaccines) are equally effective. Heptavax is no longer manufactured in the United States, and its use is restricted to hemodialysis patients and individuals who are immune compromised or have an allergy to yeast. Dosage should be in accordance with manufacturer's current recommendations.

†ISG, human immune serum globulin; HBIG, hepatitis B immune globulin.

‡A rapid immunization regimen has been approved for Engerix B in which vaccine is given immediately and at 1 and 2 months. A fourth, booster dose should be given at 12 months to achieve highest antibody titers.

Hemodynamic data in normal humans at rest (± 1 SD)

Pressure data

Right atrium		Pulmonary capillary wedge	
A wave	5 ± 3 mm Hg	A wave	8 ± 3 mm Hg
V wave	4 ± 3 mm Hg	V wave	8 ± 3 mm Hg
Mean	4 ± 2 mm Hg	Mean	7 ± 2 mm Hg

Right ventricle		Left ventricle	
Systolic	21 ± 3 mm Hg	Systolic	115 ± 11 mm Hg
End diastolic	6 ± 2 mm Hg	End diastolic	8 ± 3 mm Hg
		dP/dt_{max}	1600 ± 360 mm Hg/sec

Pulmonary artery		Aorta	
Systolic	19 ± 2 mm Hg	Systolic	115 ± 11 mm Hg
Diastolic	8 ± 2 mm Hg	Diastolic	74 ± 8 mm Hg
Mean	12 ± 2 mm Hg	Mean	93 ± 8 mm Hg

Flow data

Hemoglobin (Hb) oxygen-carrying capacity	1.36 ml/g Hb
Oxygen consumption	126 ± 24 ml/min/m^2
Arteriovenous oxygen difference	3.6 ± 0.5 vol/dl
Cardiac index	3.6 ± 0.5 L/min/m^2
Stroke index	48.0 ± 9 ml/beat/m^2
Stroke work index	0.54 ± 0.12 joules/m^2

Systemic and pulmonary vascular resistance

Total pulmonary resistance	144 ± 33 dynes-cm-sec^{-5}
Pulmonary arteriolar resistance	62 ± 29 dynes-cm-sec^{-5}
Systemic vascular resistance	1086 ± 270 dynes-cm-sec^{-5}

dP/dt_{max}, Maximum rate of rise of ventricular pressure.

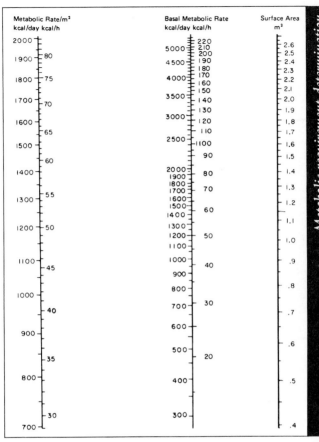

Prediction of daily metabolic requirements per square meter of body surface *(right-hand scale)* for age and sex *(left-hand scale)*. These points are connected with a straightedge, and the predicted daily or hourly requirements are read from the middle scale. (From Wilmore DW: The metabolic management of the critically ill. New York, 1977, Plenum Medical.)

Nutritional assessment

Measurement	Assessment
A. Anthropometric measurements	
1. Weight (kg)	Body weight status
2. Height (cm)	Desirable weight of adults (see Table 49-8)
3. Weight/height ratio	Body weight status
4. % Ideal body weight = $\dfrac{\text{actual weight}}{\text{ideal body weight}} \times 100$	
5. % Usual body weight = $\dfrac{\text{actual weight}}{\text{usual weight}} \times 100$	
6. % Weight change = $\dfrac{\text{usual weight} - \text{actual weight}}{\text{usual weight}} \times 100$	
7. Arm circumference (cm)	Body weight status
8. % Standard arm circumference = $\dfrac{\text{actual arm circumference}}{\text{standard arm circumference}} \times 100$	
9. Triceps skinfold (mm)	Body fatness Men: 8-23 mm Women: 10-30 mm
10. % Standard triceps skinfold = $\dfrac{\text{actual triceps skinfold}}{\text{standard triceps skinfold}} \times 100$	Lean muscle mass
11. Arm muscle circumference (mm) = arm circumference (mm) $-$ 0.314 $\times$ triceps skinfold (mm)	Midarm muscle circumference (120-140 mm)
12. % Standard arm muscle circumference = $\dfrac{\text{actual arm muscle circumference}}{\text{standard arm muscle circumference}} \times 100$	Lean muscle mass

B. Laboratory measurements
1. Total iron-binding capacity (TIBC)(μg/dl) — Labile or visceral protein status
2. Serum transferrin = $(0.8 \times TIBC) - 43$, mg/dl — Protein-calorie malnutrition / Visceral protein status
3. Serum albumin (g/dl) — Protein-calorie malnutrition / Visceral protein status / Protein-calorie malnutrition
4. White blood cell count (WBC/mm³) —
5. Total lymphocyte count = $\dfrac{\text{percent lymphocytes} \times \text{WBC}}{100}$ — Immune function
6. 24-hr urinary creatinine (mg) — Ideal urinary creatinine values (see Table 49-9)
7. Creatinine height index = $\dfrac{\text{actual urinary creatinine}}{\text{ideal urinary creatinine}} \times 100$ — Muscle or lean body mass
8. 24-hr urinary nitrogen (g) — Body protein status
9. Nitrogen balance = $\dfrac{\text{protein intake}}{6.25} - (\text{urinary urea nitrogen} + 4)$ — Body protein status
10. Basal energy expenditure — Used to derive total caloric needs
11. Complete blood count (CBC) — Anemia: Normocytic / Microcytic / Macrocytic
12. Skin tests
    Purified protein derivative (PPD) — Immune function
    Candida
    Dinitrochlorobenzene (DNCB)

Examples of commercial formulas for nutritional support

Formula	Grams per 1000 kcal			
	Protein	Fat	Carbohydrate	Lactose
Complete defined-formula diets				
Milk base: moderate residue, intact protein				
Carnation Instant Breakfast (Carnation)	55.2	27.6	124.1	84.0
Compleat (Sandoz)	40.2	40.2	119.6	24.4
Enfamil (Mead Johnson)	22.2	54.6	103.3	103.3
Meritene (Sandoz)	60.4	33.3	114.6	80.0
Sustacal (powder) (Mead Johnson)	57.0	25.9	133.3	93.0
Lactose-free, low-residue, intact protein, protein isolates				
Compleat-Modified (Sandoz)	40.1	32.0	130.8	0
Enrich (Ross)	36.1	34.8	147.3	0
Ensure (Ross)	35.1	35.1	136.8	0
Ensure HN (Ross)	41.9	33.4	133.2	0
Ensure Plus (Ross)	36.6	35.5	133.3	0
Ensure Plus HN (Ross)	41.7	33.3	133.3	0
Isocal (Mead Johnson)	32.1	41.1	126.2	0
Isocal HN (Mead Johnson)	41.5	42.4	116.0	0
Isomil (Ross)	26.4	54.4	101.5	0
Jevity (Ross)	41.9	34.7	143.1	0
Magnacal (Sherwood Medical)	35.0	40.0	125.0	0
Osmolite (Ross)	35.0	36.2	136.8	0
Osmolite HN (Ross)	41.9	34.7	133.2	0
Portagen (Mead Johnson)	34.6	47.5	114.8	0
Resource (Sandoz)	34.9	34.9	136.7	0
Prosobee (Mead Johnson)	30.0	53.0	100.0	0

Similac (Ross)	23.8	53.6	108.8	0
Sustacal (Mead Johnson)	60.3	22.8	138.6	0
Traumacal (Mead Johnson)	55.3	45.3	94.6	0
Ultracal (Mead Johnson)	41.5	42.4	116.0	0
Lactose-free, low-residue, hydrolyzed protein, amino acids				
Critical HN (Mead Johnson)	35.8	5.0	207.5	0
Nutramigen (Mead Johnson)	28.0	39.0	134.0	0
Pregestimil (Mead Johnson)	28.5	41.0	134.0	0
Reabilan (O'Brien/KMI)	31.0	39.0	131.0	0
Vital HN (Ross)	41.7	10.8	185.0	0
Vivonex T.E.N. (Sandoz)	38.2	2.8	206.0	0
Formula for special metabolic indications				
Amin-Aid (Kendall McGaw)	9.9	23.6	187.0	0
Hepatic-Aid II (Kendall McGaw)	37.5	30.8	143.3	0
Lofenalac (Mead Johnson)	32.5	39.8	129.2	0
Phenyl-Free (Mead Johnson)	50.0	16.8	162.5	0
Pulmocare (Ross)	42.0	61.3	70.7	0
Replena (Ross)	14.8	47.2	126.2	0
Travasorb Renal (Clintec)	17.1	13.3	202.7	0
Travasorb Hepatic (Clintec)	26.4	13.2	193.2	0
Supplementary feedings				
Casec (Mead Johnson)	237.6	5.4	0.0	0
Citrotein (Doyle)	60.5	2.6	184.2	0
Controlyte (Doyle)	0.0	48.0	143.0	0
MCT Oil (Mead Johnson)	0.0	120.5	0.0	0
Microlipid (Sherwood Medical)	0.0	111.0	0.0	0
Pedialyte (Ross)	0.0	0.0	250.0	0
Polycose (Ross)	0.0	0.0	250.0	0
Propac (Sherwood Medical)	189.9	20.5	0.0	0
Sumacal (Sherwood Medical)	0.0	0.0	250.0	0

Physiologic data derived from invasive monitoring

	Normal range
Cardiac index ($L/min/m^2$)	2.4-4.4
$$CI = \frac{CO}{BSA}$$	
Systemic vascular resistance ($dynes \bullet sec \bullet cm^{-5}$)	900-1400
$$SVR = \frac{MAP = CVP}{CO} \times 79.9$$	
Pulmonary vascular resistance ($dynes \bullet sec \bullet cm^{-5}$)	150-250
$$PVR = \frac{MPAP = PAWP}{CO} \times 79.9$$	
Stroke volume (ml)	
$$SV = \frac{CO}{HR}$$	
Stroke volume index (ml/m^2)	30-65
$$SVI = \frac{SV}{BSA} = \frac{CI}{HR}$$	
Left ventricular stroke work index ($g \bullet m/m^2$)	43-61
$LVSWI = SVI \times (MAP - PAOP) \times 0.0136$	
Right ventricular stroke work index ($g \bullet m/m^2$)	7-12
$RVSWI = SVI \times (MPAP - CVP) \times 0.0136$	
Oxygen content (ml/dl blood)	About 19.5
$CaO_2 = Hgb \times$ arterial O_2 saturation $\times 1.36 +$ ($PO_2 \times 0.003$)	
Arteriovenous oxygen content difference (ml/dl)	3-5
$avDO_2 = CaO_2 - CvO_2$	
Oxygen delivery (ml/min)	800-1200
O_2 delivery $= CO \times CaO_2 \times 10$	
Oxygen consumption (ml/min)	180-280
$VO_2 = CO \times (CaO_2 - CvO_2) \times 10$	
Pulmonary shunt (venoarterial admixture) (%)	<3-5%
$$\frac{QS}{Qt} = \frac{CcO_2 - CaO_2}{CcO_2 - CvO_2}$$	

Modified from Sprung CL, editor: The pulmonary artery catheter: methodology and clinical applications. Baltimore, 1983, University Park.

BSA, body surface area; CaO_2, arterial oxygen content; CcO_2, pulmonary capillary oxygen content (assumed equal to alveolar PO_2); CI, cardiac index; CO, cardiac output; CvO_2, mixed venous oxygen content; CVP, central venous pressure; Hgb, hemoglobin concentration; HR, heart rate; LVSWI, left ventricular stroke work index; MAP, mean arterial pressure; MPAP, mean pulmonary artery pressure; PAWP, pulmonary artery wedge pressure; PVR, pulmonary vascular resistance; Qs/Qt, pulmonary shunt; RVSWI, right ventricular stroke work index; SV, stroke volume; SVI, stroke volume index; SVR, systemic vascular resistance.

PROCEDURE[1] Age	20	21	22	23	24	25	26	27	28	29	30	31	32	33	34	35	36	37	38	39	40	41	42	43	44
PHYSICAL EXAMINATION																									
Blood pressure	•		•		•		•		•		•		•		•		•		•		•		•		•
Height and weight		•		•		•		•		•		•		•		•		•		•		•		•	
LAB TESTS																									
RPR[2]	•		•			•			•			•			•			•			•			•	
Gonococcal cultures[2]	•		•			•			•			•			•			•			•			•	
PPD Test[2]	•		•			•			•			•			•			•			•			•	
Thal. Sickle Tay-Sachs[3]	•		•			•			•			•			•			•			•			•	
Cholesterol					•						•					•				•					
CANCER SCREENING																									
Pelvic exam	•		•			•			•			•			•			•			•			•	
Pap Test[4]	•		•			•			•			•			•			•			•			•	
Digital rectal exam																									
Stool for occult blood																									
Mammography																					•		•		•
Breast Exam																					•	•	•	•	•
IMMUNIZATION																									
Tetanus-Diptheria	•										•										•				
Rubella[3] (Rubella Screeng)	•																			•					
Measles[6]	•																								
Mumps																									
Pneumovax																									
Influenza																									
Polio[8]	•																								
COUNSELING[9]																									

1 For patients over 70 years of age, do the same procedures at the frequency shown for patients 65 to 70 years old
2 In high-risk groups (may be performed more often if needed)
3 As part of premarital screening in high-risk groups
4 After two initial tests 1 year apart yield negative results
5 If screening test for immunity is negative
6 If born after 1956 and no prior history of immunization
7 If born after 1957 and no prior history of immunization
8 Intervention if history of inadequate immunization
9 Includes diet, smoking, exercise, alcohol, drugs, safety, safe sex, seat belts, violence, guns

Other maneuvers that might be performed at the discretion of the examiner are sigmoidoscopy, urinalysis, multichannel screening, general physical exam, thyroid screening, tonometry.
(These can be filled in blank spaces)

Health maintenance flow sheet. (From Matzen RN and Lang R: Clinical preventive medicine, St. Louis, 1993, Mosby–Yearbook. Modified from Primary Care Section, Department of Internal Medicine, Cleveland Clinic Foundation, Cleveland, Ohio.)

PROCEDURE[1] Age	45	46	47	48	49	50	51	52	53	54	55	56	57	58	59	60	61	62	63	64	65	66	67	68	69	70
PHYSICAL EXAMINATION																										
Blood Pressure		•		•		•		•		•		•		•		•		•		•		•		•		•
Height and weight		•		•		•		•		•		•		•		•		•		•		•		•		•
LAB TESTS																										
RPR[2]		•				•				•			•				•				•					
Gonococcal cultures[2]		•				•				•			•				•				•					
PPD Test[2]		•				•				•			•				•				•					
Thal., Sickle, Tay-Sachs[3]											•															
Cholesterol	•					•										•					•					•
CANCER SCREENING																										
Pelvic exam		•				•				•			•				•				•					•
Pap Test[4]		•				•				•			•				•				•					•
Digital rectal exam		•				•				•			•				•				•					•
Stool for occult blood		•		•		•		•		•		•		•		•		•		•		•		•		•
Mammography		•		•		•		•		•		•		•		•		•		•		•				
Breast Exam	•	•		•		•		•		•		•		•		•		•		•		•				
IMMUNIZATION																										
Tetanus-Diptheria						•										•										•
Rubella (Rubella Screening)																										
Measles[6]																										
Mumps[7]																										
Pneumovax																					•					
Influenza																					•	•	•	•	•	•
Polio[8]																										
COUNSELING[9]																										

1987 Revised criteria for classification of rheumatoid arthritis

1. Morning stiffness in and around the joints lasting at least 1 hour before maximal improvement.
2. At least three joint areas with simultaneous soft-tissue swelling or fluid (not bony overgrowth alone) observed by a physician. The 14 possible joint areas are right or left PIP, MCP, wrist, elbow, knee, ankle, and MTP joints.
3. At least one joint area swollen as above in a wrist, MCP, or PIP.
4. Simultaneous involvement of the same joint areas (as in 2) on both sides of the body (bilateral involvement of PIP, MCP, or MTP is acceptable without absolute symmetry).
5. Subcutaneous nodules over bony prominences, or extensor surfaces, or in juxta-articular regions, observed by a physician.
6. Demonstration of abnormal amounts of serum "rheumatoid factor" by any method that has been positive in fewer than 5% of normal control subjects.
7. Radiographic changes typical of RA on posteroanterior wrist radiographs, including erosions or unequivocal bony decalcification localized to or most marked adjacent to the involved joints (osteoarthritic changes alone do not qualify).

Arnett FC et al: 1987 revised American Rheumatism Association for classification of rheumatoid arthritis. Arthritis Rheum 31:315, 1988.

The 1982 revised criteria for the classification of systemic lupus erythematosus

Criterion	Frequency in SLE (%)
1. Malar rash	57
2. Discoid rash	18
3. Photosensitivity	43
4. Oral or nasopharyngeal ulcers	27
5. Nonerosive arthritis	86
6. Pleuritis or	52
pericarditis	18
7. Persistent proteinuria or	50
urinary casts	36
8. Seizures or	12
psychosis	13
9. Hemolytic anemia or	18
leukopenia ($<4000/mm^3$) or	46
lymphopenia ($<1500/mm^3$) or	—
thrombocytopenia ($<100,000/mm^3$)	21
10. LE cells or	73
DNA antibody or	67
Sm antibody or	31
serologic test for syphilis	15
11. Antinuclear antibody	99

Tan E et al: Arthritis Rheum 25:1271, 1982.

Systemic lupus erythematosus, criteria for diagnosis

Recommended vaccinations for international travel

Vaccine	Indications	Dose
Measles/mumps/rubella	Susceptible persons born after 1957* Contraindicated in pregnancy	One dose of combined vaccine‡
Polio		
Inactivated polio vaccine (IPV)†		
Primary series	For unimmunized adults and immunocompromised individuals. Safe in pregnancy	Three doses, 1-2 months apart
Booster series		One dose before departure
Oral polio vaccine (OPV)†		
Primary series	Not recommended in adults‡	
Booster series	For immunocompetent, immunized adults at increased risk. Safe in pregnancy	One dose before departure

Tetanus/diphtheria	
Primary series	One dose of combined vaccine at 0, 2, and 6-12 months
Booster series	One dose every 10 years
Typhoid	
Primary series	Oral vaccine: one capsule every other day for four doses
	Parenteral vaccine: 0.5 ml subcutaneously at 0 and $\geq$ 4 weeks§
	Oral vaccine: repeat primary series every 5 years
Booster series	Parenteral vaccine: 0.5 ml every 3 years

All unimmunized adults	
Travelers to developing countries, particularly rural areas where food and water sanitation are poor	

*Persons born before 1957 can be considered immune to measles and mumps; others are susceptible unless immunized or the presence of specific antibody is demonstrated. Rubella vaccine is recommended for all unvaccinated individuals without serologic evidence of previous immunity.

†The risk of adverse effects from OPV is slightly increased in adults compared with IPV. If protection is needed for these individuals within 4 weeks, however, a single dose of OPV is recommended. If protection is needed within 4 to 8 weeks, two doses of IPV 4 weeks apart are recommended; remaining dose can be administered at recommended intervals at a later time.

‡The current recommendation for measles vaccination is that two doses of vaccine be given at least 1 month apart to all persons born after 1957. Many individuals have never received the second dose and unless this can be documented, administration of measles vaccine is recommended.

§If less than 4 weeks are available before departure, 0.5 ml can be administered weekly for three doses but is slightly less effective than the standard regimen. Alternatively, the oral vaccine can be used.

ALIMENTARY TRACT FUNCTION TESTS

Gastric secretion
  Volume
    Fasting   20-100 ml/hr
    Nocturnal   <800 ml/10 hr
  Acid output (mean ± standard
    deviation)
    Basal (BAO)
      Male   3.7 ± 2.1 mEq/hr
      Female   2.2 ± 1.7 mEq/hr
    Stimulated after betazole (Hi-
      stalog), 0.5 mg/kg or pen-
      tagastrin 6 µg/kg
      subcutaneously (PAO)
      Male   23 ± 7 mEq/hr
      Female   18 ± 5 mEq/hr
    BAO/PAO ratio   <0.5
Gastrin, serum   <150 pg/ml
Gastrin, serum, following stimula-   Increases of 110 pg/ml or 100% of
  tion with intravenous secretin 2   basal level 1, 2, 5, 7, 10, 15,
  units/kg   or 30 min after secretin indicate
                                    Z-E syndrome (gastrinoma)

Intestinal absorption
  Stool fat on diet containing 80-   <8 g/24 hr
    100 g fat/day (72- to 96-hr
    collection)
  D-xylose absorption (25g
    D-xylose administered
    orally after overnight fast)
    5-hr urine collection after   >5 g
      D-xylose
    1- or 2-hr serum level after   >25 mg/dl
      D-xylose
  Triolein breath test (5 µCi ^{14}C-   >3.5% of dose/hr
    triolein administered in 30 ml
    Lipomul; breath collected
    hourly for 6 hr for measure-
    ment of breath $^{14}CO_2$)

Lactose absorption (50 g lactose administered after overnight fast; baseline and 1-, 2-, and 3-hr serum samples obtained; alternatively, breath hydrogen can be measured in expired air 90-120 min after lactose administered)

>25 mg/dl increase in serum glucose
>20 PPM H_2 in expired air

Schilling test (see Hematologic Normal Values)

Pancreatic secretion

Secretin test (2 units secretin/kg body weight, intravenously; duodenal fluid collected for 4 periods of 20 min thereafter)

Volume — >1.5 ml/kg/80 min
Bicarbonate output — >16 mEq/80 min
Bicarbonate concentration — >80 mEq/L

Bentiromide (*N*-benzoyl-L-tyrosyl-*p*-aminobenzoic acid) test (500 mg administered after overnight fast followed by oral hydration and collection of a 6-hr urine sample)

>50% urinary recovery of ingested PABA/6 hr

CARDIOVASCULAR NORMAL VALUES: Pressures

Normal pressures in the heart and great vessels*

Pressures	Average (mm Hg)	Range (mm Hg)	Pressures	Average (mm Hg)	Range (mm Hg)
Right atrium			Left atrium		
Mean	2.8	1-5	Mean	7.9	2-12
a wave	5.6	2.5-7.0	a wave	10.4	4-16
z point	2.9	1.5-5.0	z point	7.6	1-13
c wave	3.8	1.5-6.0	v wave	12.8	6-21
x wave	1.7	0-5	Left ventricle		
v wave	4.6	2.0-7.5	Peak systolic	130	90-140
y wave	2.4	0-6	End diastolic	8.7	5-12
Right ventricle			Brachial artery		
Peak systolic	25	17-32	Mean	85	70-105
End diastolic	4	1-7	Peak systolic	130	90-140
Pulmonary artery			End diastolic	70	60-90
Mean	15	9-19			
Peak systolic	25	17-32			
End diastolic	9	4-13			
Pulmonary artery wedge					
Mean	9	4.5-13.0			

*Reference elevation = 10 cm above the spine of the recumbent subject.

Cardiovascular Function Tests

Cardiac index

$$L/min/m^2 = \frac{CO}{\text{body surface area (BSA)}}$$

Normal = 2.8-4.2

Cardiac output

$CO = \text{heart rate} \times \text{stroke volume}$

Cardiac output (Fick principle)

$$CO \text{ (L/min)} = \frac{O_2 \text{ consumption (ml } O_2/\text{min)}}{AV\ O_2 \text{ difference (ml } O_2/\text{L)}}$$

where

O_2 consumption (basal state estimate) = 3 ml O_2/min/kg body weight

AV O_2 difference = arterial O_2 content − venous O_2 content (ml O_2/L)

O_2 content (ml/dl) = Hb (g/dl) × 1.39 (ml O_2/g Hb) × % saturation

O_2 content (ml O_2/L) = ml/dl × 10

Therefore

$$CO \text{ (L/min)} = \frac{3 \text{ (ml/min)} \times \text{weight (kg)}}{(SaO_2 - S\bar{v}O_2)\ (1.39) \times \text{Hb (g/dl)} \times 10}$$

Mean arterial pressure

Mean arterial pressure = diastolic pressure
$\qquad\qquad\qquad\qquad\quad$ + ⅓ (systolic pressure − diastolic pressure)

Resistance—can be expressed in absolute resistance units (ARU) of dyne-sec-cm^{-5} or hybrid resistance units (HRU) of mm Hg/L/min; ARU = 80 HRU

Systemic vascular resistance (SVR)

$$SVR = \frac{\overline{SA} - \overline{RA}}{CO} \text{ (Normal = 1130 dyne-sec-cm}^{-5} \pm 178)$$

Pulmonary arteriolar resistance (PAR)

$$PAR = \frac{\overline{PA} - \overline{LA}}{CO} \text{ (Normal = 67 dyne-sec-cm}^{-5} \pm 23)$$

Total pulmonary resistance (TPR)

$$TPR = \frac{\overline{PA}}{CO} \text{ (Normal = 205 dyne-sec-cm}^{-5} \pm 51)$$

Total systemic resistance (TSR)

$$TSR = \frac{\overline{SA}}{CO}$$

where

$\overline{RA}$ = mean right atrial pressure

$\overline{PA}$ = mean pulmonary artery pressure

$\overline{LA}$ = mean left atrial pressure

$\overline{SA}$ = mean systemic arterial pressure

CO = cardiac output

CEREBROSPINAL FLUID NORMAL VALUES

Bilirubin	0
Cells	0-5/mm^3, all lymphocytes
Chloride	110-129 mEq/L
Glucose	48-86 mg/dl or ≥60% of serum glucose
pH	7.34-7.43
Pressure	7-20 cm water
Protein, lumbar	15-45 mg/dl
Albumin	58%
α_1-globulins	9%
α_2-globulins	8%
β-globulins	10%
γ-globulins	10 (5-12)%
Protein, cisternal	15-25 mg/dl
Protein, ventricular	5-15 mg/dl

ENDOCRINOLOGIC NORMAL VALUES
Hormone and Metabolite Normal Values

Adrenocorticotropin (ACTH), serum	15-100 pg/ml
Aldosterone (mean ± standard deviation)	
Serum	
210 mEq/day sodium diet	
Supine	48 ± 29 pg/ml
Upright (2 hr)	65 ± 23 pg/ml
110 mEq/day sodium diet	
Supine	107 ± 45 pg/ml
Upright (2 hr)	532 ± 228 pg/ml
Urine	5-19 μg/24 hr
Calcitonin, serum	
Basal	0.15-0.35 ng/ml
Stimulated	<0.6 ng/ml
Catecholamines, free urinary	<110 μg/24 hr
Chorionic gonadotropin, serum	
Pregnancy	
First month	10-10,000 mIU/ml
Second and third months	10,000-100,000 mIU/ml
Second trimester	10,000-30,000 mIU/ml
Third trimester	5000-15,000 mIU/ml
Nonpregnant	<3 mIU/ml
Cortisol	
Serum	
8 AM	5-25 μg/dl
8 PM	<10 μg/dl
Cosyntropin stimulation (30-90 min after 0.25 mg cosyntropin intramuscularly or intravenously)	>10 μg/dl rise over baseline
Overnight suppression (8 AM serum cortisol after 1 mg dexamethasone orally at 11 PM)	≤5 μg/dl
Urine	20-70 μg/24 hr

Hormone and Metabolite Normal Values—cont'd

C-peptide, serum	0.28-0.63 pmol/ml	
11-Deoxycortisol, serum		
Basal	0-1.4 µg/dl	
Metyrapone stimulation (30 mg/kg orally 8 hr prior to level)	>7.5 µg/dl	
Epinephrine, plasma	<35 pg/ml	
Estradiol, serum		
Male	20-50 pg/ml	
Female	25-200 pg/ml	
Estrogens, urine (increased during pregnancy; decreased after menopause)	*Male*	*Female*
Total	4-25 µg/24 hr	5-100 µg/24 hr
Estriol	1-11 µg/24 hr	0-65 µg/24 hr
Estradiol	0-6 µg/24 hr	0-14 µg/24 hr
Estrone	3-8 µg/24 hr	4-31 µg/24 hr
Etiocholanolone, serum	<1.2 µg/dl	
Follicle-stimulating hormone, serum		
Male	2-18 mIU/ml	
Female		
Follicular phase	5-20 mIU/ml	
Peak midcycle	30-50 mIU/ml	
Luteal phase	5-15 mIU/ml	
Postmenopausal	>50 mIU/ml	
Free thyroxine index, serum	1-4 ng/dl	
Gastrin, serum (fasting)	30-200 pg/ml	
Growth hormone, serum		
Adult, fasting	<5 ng/ml	
Glucose load (100 g orally)	<5 ng/ml	
Levodopa stimulation (500 mg orally in a fasting state)	>5 ng/ml rise over baseline within 2 hr	
17-Hydroxycorticosteroids, urine		
Male	2-12 mg/24 hr	
Female	2-8 mg/24 hr	
5'-Hydroxyindoleacetic acid (5'-HIAA), urine	2-9 mg/24 hr	
Insulin, plasma		
Fasting	6-20 µU/ml	
Hypoglycemia (serum glucose <50 mg/dl)	<5 µU/ml	
17-Ketosteroids, urine		
Under 8 years old	0-2 mg/24 hr	
Adolescent	0-18 mg/24 hr	
Adult		
Male	8-18 mg/24 hr	
Female	5-15 mg/24 hr	
Luteinizing hormone, serum		
Male adult	2-18 mIU/ml	
Female adult		
Basal	5-22 mIU/ml	
Ovulation	30-250 mIU/ml	
Postmenopausal	>30 mIU/ml	

Metanephrines, urine	<1.3 mg/24 hr
Norepinephrine	
Plasma	150-450 pg/ml
Urine	<100 μg/24 hr
Parathyroid hormone, serum	
C-terminal	150-350 pg/ml
N-terminal	230-630 pg/ml
Pregnanediol, urine	
Female	
Follicular phase	<1.5 mg/24 hr
Luteal phase	2.0-4.2 mg/24 hr
Postmenopausal	0.2-1.0 mg/24 hr
Male	<1.5 mg/24 hr
Progesterone, serum	
Female	
Follicular phase	0.02-0.9 ng/ml
Luteal phase	6-30 ng/ml
Male	<2 ng/ml
Prolactin, serum	
Nonpregnant	
Day	5-25 ng/ml
Night	20-40 ng/ml
Pregnant	150-200 ng/ml
Radioactive iodine (^{131}I) uptake (RAIU)	5%-25% at 24 hr (varies with iodine intake)
Renin activity, plasma (mean ± standard deviation)	
Normal diet	
Supine	1.1 ± 0.8 ng/ml/hr
Upright	1.9 ± 1.7 ng/ml/hr
Low-sodium diet	
Supine	2.7 ± 1.8 ng/ml/hr
Upright	6.6 ± 2.5 ng/ml/hr
Diuretics and low-sodium diet	10.0 ± 3.7 ng/ml/hr
Testosterone, total plasma	
Bound	
Adolescent male	<100 ng/dl
Adult male	300-1100 ng/dl
Female	25-90 ng/dl
Unbound	
Adult male	3-24 ng/dl
Female	0.09-1.30 ng/dl
Thyroid-stimulating hormone, serum	<10 μU/ml
Thyroxine (T_4), serum	
Total	4-11 μg/dl
Free	0.8-2.4 ng/dl
Thyroxine-binding globulin capacity, serum	15-25 μg T_4/dl
Thyroxine index, free	1-4 ng/dl
Tri-iodothyronine (T_3), serum	70-190 ng/dl
T_3 resin uptake	25%-45%
Vanillylmandelic acid (VMA), urine	1-8 mg/24 hr

Endocrine Function Tests

Adrenal gland

Glucocorticoid suppression: overnight dexamethasone suppression test (8 AM serum cortisol after 1 mg dexamethasone orally at 11 PM) — ≤5 µg/dl

Glucocorticoid stimulation: cosyntropin stimulation test (serum cortisol 30-90 min after 0.25 mg cosyntropin intramuscularly or intravenously) — >10 µg/ml more than baseline serum cortisol

Metyrapone test, single dose (8 AM serum deoxycortisol after 30 mg/kg metyrapone orally at midnight) — >7.5 µg/dl

Aldosterone suppression: sodium depletion test (urine aldosterone collected on day 3 of 200 mEq day/sodium diet) — <20 µg/24 hr

Pancreas

Glucose tolerance test* serum glucose after 100 g glucose orally)

60 min after ingestion	<180 mg/dl
90 min after ingestion	<160 mg/dl
120 min after ingestion	<125 mg/dl

Pituitary gland

Adrenocorticotropic hormone (ACTH) stimulation. See Adrenal gland, Metyrapone test

Growth hormone stimulation: insulin tolerance test (serum growth hormone after 0.1 U/kg regular insulin intravenously after an overnight fast to induce a 50% fall in serum glucose concentration or symptomatic hypoglycemia) — >5 ng/ml rise over baseline

Levodopa test (serum growth hormone after 0.5 g levodpoa orally while fasting) — >5 ng/ml rise over baseline within 2 hr

Growth hormone suppression: glucose tolerance test (serum growth hormone after 100 g glucose orally after 8 hr fast) — <5 ng/ml within 2 hr

---

*Add 10 mg/dl for each decade over 50 years of age.

Luteinizing hormone (LH) stimulation: gonadotropin-releasing hormone (GnRH) test (serum LH after 100 μg GnRH intravenously or intramuscularly)	4- to 6-fold rise over baseline
Thyroid-stimulating hormone (TSH) stimulation: thyrotropin-releasing hormone (TRH) stimulation test (serum TSH after 400 μg TRH intraveneously)	>2-fold rise over baseline within 2 hr

Thyroid gland

Radioactive iodine uptake (RAIU) suppression test (RAIU on day 7 after 25 μg tri-iodothyronine orally 4 times daily)	<10% to <50% baseline
Thyrotropin-releasing hormone (TRH) stimulation test. See Pituitary gland, Thyroid-stimulating hormone (TSH) stimulation	

HEMATOLOGIC NORMAL VALUES

Differential cell count of bone marrow

Myeloid cells	
Neutrophilic series	
Myeloblasts	0.3%-5.0%
Promyelocytes	1%-8%
Myelocytes	5%-19%
Metamyelocytes	9%-24%
Bands	9%-15%
Segmented cells	7%-30%
Eosinophil precursors	0.5%-3.0%
Eosinophils	0.5%-4.0%
Basophilic series	0.2%-0.7%
Erythroid cells	
Pronormoblasts	1%-8%
Basophilic normoblasts	
Polychromatophilic normoblasts	7%-32%
Orthochromatic normoblasts	
Megakaryocytes	0.1%
Lymphoreticular cells	
Lymphocytes	3%-17%
Plasma cells	0%-2%
Reticulum cells	0.1%-2.0%
Monocytes	0.5%-5.0%
Myeloid/erythroid ratio	0.6-2.7

HEMATOLOGIC NORMAL VALUES—cont'd

Acid hemolysis test (Ham)	No hemolysis
Carboxyhemoglobin	
Nonsmoker	<1%
Smoker	2.1%-4.2%
Cold hemolysis test	No hemolysis
(Donath-Landsteiner)	
Complete blood count (see Table 3)	
Erythrocyte life span	
Normal	120 days
^{51}Cr-labeled half-life	28 days
Erythropoietin by radioimmunassay	9-33 mU/dl
Ferritin, serum	
Male	15-200 µg/L
Female	12-150 µg/L
Folate, RBC	120-670 ng/ml
Fragility, osmotic	
Hemolysis begins 0.45%-0.38% NaCl	
Hemolysis completed 0.33%-0.30% NaCl	
Haptoglobin, serum	100-300 mg/dl
Hemoglobin	
Hemoglobin A_{1c}	0%-5% of total
Hemoglobin A_2 by column	2%-3% of total
Hemoglobin, fetal	<1% of total
Hemoglobin, plasma	0%-5% of total
Hemoglobin, serum	2-3 mg/ml
Iron, serum	
Male	75-175 µg/dl
Female	65-165 µg/dl
Iron-binding capacity, total serum (TIBC)	250-450 µg/dl
Iron turnover rate (plasma)	20-42 mg/24 hr
Leukocyte alkaline phosphatase (LAP) score	30-150
Methemoglobin	<1.8%
Reticulocytes (see Table 3)	
Schilling test (urinary excretion of radiolabeled vitamin B_{12} after "flushing" intramuscular injection of B_{12})	6%-30% of oral dose within 24 hr

Sedimentation rate	*Male*	*Female*
Wintrobe	0-5 mm/hr	0-15 mm/hr
Westergren	0-15 mm/hr	0-20 mm/hr

Transferrin saturation, serum	20%-50%	

Volume	*Male*	*Female*
Blood	52-83 ml/kg	50-75 ml/kg
Plasma	25-43 ml/kg	28-45 ml/kg
Red cell	20-36 ml/kg	19-31 ml/kg

Complete blood count

Parameter	Male	Female
Hematocrit (%)	40-52	38-48
Hemoglobin (g/dl)	13.5-18.0	12-16
Erythrocyte count ($\times 10^{12}$ cells/L)	4.6-6.2	4.2-5.4
Reticulocyte count (%)	0.6-2.6	0.4-2.4
MCV (fL)	82-98	82-98
MCH (pg)	27-32	27-32
MCHC (g/dl)	32-36	32-36
WBC ($\times 10^9$ cells/L)	4.5-11.0	4.5-11.0
Segmented neutrophils	1.8-7.7	1.8-7.7
Average (%)	40-60	40-60
Bands (cells)	0-0.3	0-0.3
Average (%)	0-3	0-3
Eosinophils (cells $\times 10^9$/L)	0-0.5	0-0.5
Average (%)	0-5	0-5
Basophils (cells $\times 10^9$/L)	0-0.2	0-0.2
Average (%)	0-1	0-1
Lymphocytes (cells $\times 10^9$/L)	1.0-4.8	1.0-4.8
Average (%)	20-45	20-45
Monocytes (cells $\times 10^9$/L)	0-0.8	0-0.8
Average (%)	2-6	2-6
Platelet count (cells $\times 10^9$/L)	150-350	150-350

Coagulation Normal Values

Template bleeding time	3.5-7.5 min
Clot retraction, qualitative	Apparent in 30-60 min; complete in 24 hr, usually in 6 hr
Coagulation time (Lee-White)	
Glass tubes	5-15 min
Siliconized tubes	20-60 min
Euglobulin lysis time	120-240 min
Factors II, V, VII, VIII, IX, X, XI, or XII	100% or 1.0 unit/ml
Fibrin degradation products	<10 µg/ml or titer ≤1.4
Fibrinogen	200-400 mg/ml
Partial thromboplastin time, activated	20-40 sec
Prothrombin time (PT)	11-14 sec
Thrombin time	10-15 sec
Whole blood clot lysis time	>24 hr

PULMONARY FUNCTION TESTS

Abbreviations
P_B = barometric pressure (mm Hg)
FiO_2 = inspired oxygen fraction (0.21 = room air)
$PaCO_2$ = partial pressure of carbon dioxide in arterial blood (mm Hg)
$PACO_2$ = partial pressure of carbon droxide in alveolar gas (mm Hg)
$PaOO_2$ = partial pressure of oxygen in arterial blood (mm Hg)
PAO_2 = partial pressure of oxygen in alveolar gas (mm Hg)

Alveolar-arterial oxygen gradient ($FiO_2 = 0.21$)
P(A-a) in adolescents = <10 mm Hg
    adults <40 years = 10 mm Hg
        >40 years = 10-15 mm Hg

Alveolar oxygen partial pressure (sea level, $FiO_2 = 0.21$)
    $PAO_2 = 150 - (1.2 \times PaCO_2)$

Blood gases ($FiO_2 = 0.21$)

	Arterial	*Alveolar*
PO_2	80-105 mm Hg	90-115 mm Hg
PCO_2	38-44 mm Hg	38-44 mm Hg
pH	7.35-7.45	

Spirometric volumes and lung volumes are size-dependent.
Typical normal values for adults are provided.

Lung volumes	*Male*	*Female*
Total lung capacity (TLC)	6-7 L	5-6 L
Functional residual capacity (FRC)	2-3 L	2-3 L
Residual values (RV)	1-2 L	1-2 L
Measures of air flow		
Forced vital capacity (FVC)	4.0 L	3.0 L
1 sec forced vital capacity (FEV_1)	>3.0 L	>2.0 L
Pulmonary resistance (RL)	<3.0 cm H_2O/sec/L	
Airway resistance (Raw)	<2.5 cm H_2O/sec/L	
Other		
Pulmonary compliance (CL)	0.2 L/cm H_2O	
Diffusing capacity (DLCO)	25 ml CO/min/mm Hg	

RENAL FUNCTION TESTS

Anion gap

$Na^+ - HCO_3^- + Cl^- = 12 \pm 2$ mEq/L

Osmolality

Osmolality (serum) $= 2$ Na (mEq/L) $+ \dfrac{BUN\ (mg/dl)}{2.8} + \dfrac{glucose\ (mg/dl)}{18}$

Bicarbonate deficit

HCO_3^- deficit $=$ body weight (kg) $\times 0.4$ (desired HCO_3^- $-$ observed HCO_3^-)

Glomerular filtration rate

$$GFR = \frac{Ucr \times V}{Pcr}$$

$\quad = 130 \pm 20$ ml/min in males

$\quad = 120 \pm 15$ ml/min in females

$\quad \cong \dfrac{Ucr}{Pcr} \times 70$

where
Ucr $=$ urine creatinine (mg/dl)
Pcr $=$ plasma creatinine (mg/dl)
V $=$ urine volume/24 hr (ml/min)

Renal plasma flow

$$RPF = \frac{Upah \times V}{Ppah}$$

$\quad = 700 \pm 130$ ml/min in males

$\quad = 600 \pm 100$ ml/min in females

where
Upah $=$ urine para-aminohippuric acid (mg/dl)
V $=$ urine volume/24 hr (ml/min)
Ppah $=$ plasma para-aminohippuric acid (mg/dl)

SEMEN NORMAL VALUES

Liquefaction	Complete in 15 min
Morphology	>50% normal forms
Motility	>75% motile forms
pH	7.2-8.0
Spermatocrit	10%
Spermatocyte count	>50 million/ml
Volume	2.0-6.6 ml

SERUM NORMAL VALUES

Acetoacetate	0.3-2.0 mg/dl
Acid phosphatase	0-0.8 U/ml
Acid phosphatase, prostatic	2.5-12.0 IU/L
Albumin	3.0-5.5 g/dl
Aldolase	1-6 IU/L
Alkaline phosphatase	
15-20 years	40-200 IU/L
20-101 years	35-125 IU/L
Alpha-1 antitrypsin	200-500 mg/dl
ALT	0-40 IU/L
Ammonia	11-35 μmol/L
Amylase, serum	2-20 U/L
Anion gap	8-12 mEq/L (mmol/L)
Ascorbic acid	0.4-1.5 mg/dl
AST	5-40 IU/L
Bilirubin	
Total	0.2-1.2 mg/dl
Direct	0-0.4 mg/dl
Calcium, serum	8.7-10.6 mg/dl
Carbon dioxide, total	18-30 mEq/L (mmol/L)
Carcinoembryonic antigen, serum	<2.5 μg/L
Carotene (carotenoids)	50-300 μg/dl
C3 complement	55-120 mg/dl
C4 complement	14-51 mg/dl
Ceruloplasmin	15-60 mg/dl
Chloride, serum	95-105 mEq/L (mmol/L)
Cholesterol, total	
12-19 years	120-230 mg/dl
20-29 years	120-240 mg/dl
30-39 years	140-270 mg/dl
40-49 years	150-310 mg/dl
50-59 years	160-330 mg/dl
Copper	100-200 μg/dl
Creatine kinase, total	20-200 IU/L
Creatine kinase, isoenzymes	
MM fraction	94%-95%
MB fraction	0%-5%
BB fraction	0%-2%
Normal values in	
Heart	80% MM, 20% MB
Brain	100% BB
Skeletal, muscle	95% MM, 2% MB
Creatinine, serum	
Female adult	0.5-1.3 mg/dl
Male adult	0.7-1.5 mg/dl
Delta-aminolevulinic acid (ALA)	<200 μg/dl
α-Fetoprotein, serum	<40 μg/L
Folate, serum	1.9-14.0 ng/ml
Gamma glutamyl transpeptidase	
Male	12-38 IU/L
Female	9-31 IU/L
Gastrin	150 pg/ml
Glucose, serum (fasting)	70-115 mg/dl
Glucose-6-phosphate dehydrogenase	5-10 IU/g Hb
G6PD screen, qualitative	Negative
Haptoglobin	100-300 mg/dl
Hemoglobin A_2	0%-4% of total Hb
Hemoglobin F	0%-2% of total Hb

Immunoglobulin, quantitation	
IgG	700-1500 mg/dl
IaA	70-400 mg/dl
IgM	
Male	30-250 mg/dl
Female	30-300 mg/dl
IgD	0-40 mg/dl
Insulin, fasting	6-20 μU/ml
Iron-binding capacity	250-400 μg/dl
Iron, total, serum	40-150 μg/dl
Lactic acid	0.6-1.8 mEq/L
LDH, serum	20-220 IU/L
LDH isoenzymes	
LDH_1	20%-34%
LDH_2	28%-41%
LDH_3	15%-25%
LDH_4	3%-12%
LDH_5	6%-15%
Leucine aminopeptidase (LAP)	30-55 IU/L
Lipase	4-24 IU/dl
Magnesium, serum	1.5-2.5 mEq/L
5'-Nucleotidase	0.3-3.2 Bodansky units
Osmolality, serum	278-305 mOsm/kg serum water
Phenylalanine	3 mg/dl
Phosphorus, inorganic, serum	2.0-4.3 mg/dl
Potassium, plasma	3.1-4.3 mEq/L
Potassium, serum	3.5-5.2 mEq/L
Protein, total, serum	
2-55 years	5.0-8.0 g/dl
55-101 years	6.0-8.3 g/dl
Protein electrophoresis, serum	
Albumin	3.2-5.2 g/dl
Alpha-1	0.6-1.0 g/dl
Alpha-2	0.6-1.0 g/dl
Beta	0.6-1.2 g/dl
Gamma	0.7-1.5 g/dl
Sodium, serum	135-145 mEq/L
Sulfate	0.5-1.5 mg/dl
T_3 uptake	25%-45%
T_4	4-11 μg/dl
Triglycerides	
2-29 years	10-140 mg/dl
30-39 years	20-150 mg/dl
40-49 years	20-160 mg/dl
50-59 years	20-190 mg/dl
60-101 years	20-200 mg/dl
Urea nitrogen, serum	
2-65 years	5-22 mg/dl
Male	10-38 mg/dl
Female	8-26 mg/dl
Uric acid	
10-59 years	
Male	2.5-9.0 mg/dl
Female	2.0-8.0 mg/dl
60-101 years	
Male	2.5-9.0 mg/dl
Female	2.5-9.0 mg/dl
Viscosity	1.4-1.8 (serum compared to H_2O)
Vitamin A	0.15-0.60 μg/ml
Vitamin B_{12}	200-850 pg/ml

STOOL NORMAL VALUES

Bulk
  Wet weight   <197 g/24 hr
  Dry weight   <66.4 g/24 hr
Coproporphyrin   12-832 mg/24 hr
Fat   <7.2 g/24 hr
Nitrogen   <2.2 g/24 hr
Urobilinogen   40-280 mg/24 hr
Water   Approximately 65%

SYNOVIAL FLUID NORMAL VALUES

Cells	<200 cells/mm^3
Polymorphonuclear cells	<25%
Crystals	None
Fibrin clot	None
Glucose	Same as serum
Hyaluronic acid	2.45-3.97 g/L
pH	7.31-7.64
Protein	<2.5 g/dl
Albumin	63%
α_1-Globulins	7%
α_2-Globulins	7%
β-Globulins	9%
γ-Globulins	14%
Relative viscosity	High
Uric acid	Same as serum

TOXICOLOGY

Serum values for drugs and toxic substances

Substance	Therapeutic range	Toxic range
Acetaminophen	10-20 mg/L	>150 mg/L 5 hr after ingestion
Alcohol	0	150-300 mg/dl: confusion
		300-450 mg/dl: stupor
		>400 mg/dl: coma → death
Amphetamine	0	
Amobarbital	7-15 μg/ml	
Bromide	20-120 mg/dl	>150 mg/dl
Carbamazepine	6-10 μg/ml	
Clonazepam	0.02-0.10 μg/ml	
Digitoxin	5-40 ng/ml	
Digoxin	0.5-2.0 ng/ml	Clinically determined
Diphenylhydantoin	10-20 μg/ml	
Ethosuximide	40-100 μg/ml	
Glutethimide	1-7 μg/ml	
Lead	occupational >80 μg/dl	
Lithium	0.5-1.5 mEq/L	2.0 mEq/L
Meprobamate	10-20 μg/ml	30-70 μg/ml: coma
Methanol	0	
Pentobarbital	4-6 μg/ml	
Phenobarbital	5-30 μg/ml	>40 μg/ml
Primidone	4-12 μg/ml	
Procainamide	4-6 μg/ml	
Propranolol	50-100 ng/ml	
Quinidine	3-5 μg/ml	>8 μg/ml
Salicylate	200-250 mg/L	300 mg/L
Secobarbital	3-5 μg/ml	
Theophylline	10-20 μg/ml	
Valproic acid	<100 μg/ml	

Normal values of standard laboratory and function tests

URINE NORMAL VALUES

Acidity, titratable	20-40 mEq/24 hr
Ammonia	30-50 mEq/24 hr
Amylase	35-260 Somogyi units/hr
Bence Jones protein	None detected
Bilirubin	None detected
Calcium	
Unrestricted diet	<300 mg/24 hr (men)
	<250 mg/24 hr (women)
Low-calcium diet (200 mg/day for 3 days)	<150 mg/24 hr
Chloride	120-240 mEq/24 hr (varies with dietary intake)
Copper	0-32 μg/24 hr
Creatine	
Male	0-40 mg/24 hr
Female	0-100 mg/24 hr
Creatinine	1.0-1.6 g/24 hr or 15-25 mg/kg body weight/24 hr
Cysteine, qualitative	Negative
Delta-aminolevulinic acid	1.3-7.0 mg/24 hr
Glucose	
Qualitative	None detected
Quantitative	16-300 mg/24 hr
Hemoglobin	None detected
Homogentisic acid	None detected
Iron	40-140 μg/24 hr
Lead	0-120 μg/24 hr
Myoglobin	None detected
Osmolality	50-1200 mOsm/L
pH	4.6-8.0
Phenylpyruvic acid, qualitative	None detected
Phosphorus	0.8-2.0 g/24 hr
Porphobilinogen	
Qualitative	None detected
Quantitative	0-2.4 mg/24 hr
Porphyrins	
Coproporphyrin	50-250 μg/24 hr
Uroporphyrin	10-30 μg/24 hr
Potassium	25-100 mEq/24 hr
Protein	
Qualitative	None detected
Quantitative	10-150 mg/24 hr
Sodium	130-260 mEq/24 hr (varies with dietary sodium intake)
Specific gravity	1.003-1.030
Uric acid	80-976 mg/24 hr
Urobilinogen	0.05-3.5 mg/24 hr <1.0 Ehrlich units/2 hr

Admitting _____

Anesthesia _____

CCU _____

ECG _____

EEG _____

ER _____

ICU _____

Information _____

IV Team _____

Laboratory _____

   Chemistry _____

   Hematology _____

   Microbiology _____

   Other _____

Medical Records _____

Nuclear Medicine _____

Paging _____

Pathology _____

Pharmacy _____

Physical Therapy _____

Pulmonary Function _____

Radiology _____

Recovery Room _____

Respiratory Therapy _____

Security _____

Social Service _____

Sonography _____

Other _____

Nursing Stations

_____   _____
_____   _____
_____   _____
_____   _____

House Staff

_____   _____
_____   _____
_____   _____
_____   _____
_____   _____
_____   _____
_____   _____
_____   _____
_____   _____
_____   _____
_____   _____

Attending Staff

_____   _____
_____   _____
_____   _____
_____   _____
_____   _____
_____   _____
_____   _____
_____   _____
_____   _____
_____   _____
_____   _____
_____   _____
_____   _____
_____   _____
_____   _____

A

I